HISTORY *of the* SCHOOL OF NURSING
of the MONTREAL GENERAL HOSPITAL

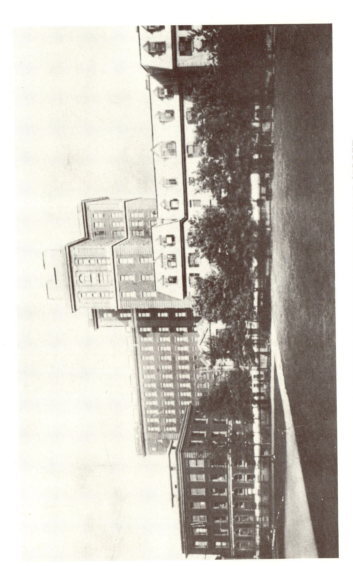

THE OLD HOSPITAL BUILDINGS ON DORCHESTER STREET
The original building is in front, on the right.

HISTORY *of*
the SCHOOL OF NURSING *of*
the MONTREAL GENERAL
HOSPITAL

By

H. E. MacDermot, M.D., F.R.C.P.(C.)

THE
ALUMNAE ASSOCIATION
MONTREAL
1940

PRINTED IN CANADA BY
THE SOUTHAM PRINTING COMPANY LIMITED
MONTREAL DIVISION

PREFACE

The alteration in the name of the School from "School for Nurses" to "School of Nursing" has led to a corresponding change in the title of its History.

The book has long been out of print and the Alumnae have decided to make it again available; partly to bring it up to date, and also through it to pay tribute to the memory of Miss Norena Mackenzie, an outstanding teacher in the School for several years, and internationally recognized for her devotion to nursing.

A short commentary on developments in the School has been added. Chief amongst these has been the transfer of the Hospital and its School from outmoded and (as they had come to be) poorly situated habitations, to entirely new buildings in an impressive and readily accessible environment. This was a major undertaking; it called for prolonged and intensive effort, both in preparation and execution, and its consummation brought about far-reaching physical and psychological benefits to the institution.

The additional material follows as a direct continuation of the original History, and the appendices appear, as before, at the end of the book. The main change in these is in the lists of the graduates. The extremely laborious work involved in bringing this valuable record up to date has been done entirely by Miss M. I. MacLeod.

My thanks are due to Mrs. Isobel MacLeod, Director, her Associates Miss Martha MacDonald, Miss Blanche Herman and Miss Anna Christie, and to Mrs. B. S. Johnston, for their ever-ready response to my many inquiries. Mr. A. H. Westbury has also kindly read the manuscript.

H. E. MacDermot

April, 1961.

i

INTRODUCTION

The preparation of this history began in 1938. At that time, plans were being made for a celebration of the fiftieth anniversary of the founding of the School, in 1940, and it was thought that a short sketch of its history would form an appropriate memorial booklet.

It was soon found, however, that a history of the School deserved more space than would be given a mere sketch. The School not only has a history of its own, but it is linked up with the Montreal General Hospital, which is possessed of its own striking story. The background for the development of nursing in Montreal had to be considered. The sketch, therefore, grew into a volume.

The outbreak of war altered the plans for the celebration of the anniversary. These eventually took the form of a special meeting of the Alumnae Association held on the anniversary of Miss Livingston's arrival at the hospital, which was made the occasion for reminiscences by a great many of the older graduates of the School. An account of this has been included.

The book is being published by the Alumnae Association, with very generous assistance from the Governors of the hospital.

The founder of the School, Miss Nora Livingston, occupies a dominating position in its story, and rightly so. But no attempt has been made to give a full account of herself. A description of what she did is the most eloquent tribute to her, and her character stands out in her work. It was felt, also, that the extracts from her letters, published separately, would give some impression of her quick, decisive mind, with its shrewdness of judgment, much better than any formal description.

Thanks are due for help and information from a great many friends of the Hospital and School. Dr. E. M. Eberts, one of Miss Livingston's closest friends, the Rev. Arthur French and Dr. Maude Abbott, have been particularly helpful.

HISTORY *of the* SCHOOL OF NURSING
of the MONTREAL GENERAL HOSPITAL

CHAPTER I

The history of a training school for nurses cannot be entirely separated from the general history of the hospital to which it is attached. So that some account of the growth of the Montreal General Hospital will be necessary in describing the development of its training school.

The Montreal General Hospital has sprung from very unostentatious beginnings. The first "quickening" of the hospital showed itself in the work of the Female Benevolent Society of Montreal. This was an organization formed in 1816 to deal with poverty and illness in the city. The Hôtel Dieu with its fine record dating back to 1644 was insufficient for the needs of the rapidly growing community.

Among the activities of the Female Benevolent Society was the opening in 1818 of a small hospital of four beds in Chaboillez Square, bearing the pleasant title of "The House of Recovery".[1] This very soon showed the need for something on a larger scale, and in 1819 a group of business men took charge of the hospital and bought a house on Craig Street, which they equipped with 24 beds, the military authorities providing the bedding. There was a staff of four medical gentlemen and quarterly reports were issued. It was now called "The Montreal General Hospital". The medical work had from the first been done by the "medical faculty" of the city, who were very graciously thanked in the *Montreal Gazette* by Mrs. Benaiah Gibb, the directress of the Benevolent Society.

This building too was soon outgrown by its needs, and in 1820 a group of prominent citizens bought the land on which the present

---

[1] This was looked after by the "Committee of the Soup Kitchen", which therefore may be regarded as the progenitor of the Committee of Management of the hospital.

building stands. This site in the French regime had formed part of the outer defences of Montreal, being occupied by the strong-point known as "La Redoute de l'Enfant Jésu".([1]) The first building of the institution was erected in 1822 and the hospital opened its doors for patients on May 3, 1823. Eight patients were brought up from the establishment on Craig Street, but the first patient recorded as being admitted was one Richard King, "from La Chine, with hepatitis, recommended by La Chine Canal Company, and to pay 5/ per week." The construction of the Lachine Canal had been begun in the previous year, and it provided a good many cases for the hospital, under such diagnoses as "fractura", "vulnus", "contusio", and "ambustio" (burns).

From the very beginning there was a great variety of nationalities amongst the hospital population. Within a few days the admission book records "Hibernus, Anglus, Americanus, Germanicus, Canadensis, Scotus, Norwegian and Welshman." The last two do not seem to have been thought worthy of Latin appellations! Hibernus (usually shortened to "Hib.") was the most frequent entry, on account of the large numbers of Irish immigrants at that time.

The original plan of the hospital called for a central building of two stories, with a basement and attic, 76 by 40 feet, and a capacity of 72 beds. It was provided that as circumstances allowed, two wings were to be added, each with a further capacity of 72 beds. Circumstances were duly obliging, and in 1832, the east or Richardson wing was added, and the west, or Reid wing in 1848. If the hospital were to be called by any other name none would be more appropriate than that of the Honourable John Richardson. He, with Wm. McGillivray and Samuel Gerrard, had bought the site. He was the first president of the hospital and it was he who paid off the debt when it was found that the building cost nearly double the original estimate. The Reid wing was a memorial to Chief Justice Reid by his widow.

The medical staff consisted of four men; John Stephenson, William Robertson, A. F. Holmes and William Caldwell, all Edin-

([1]) In 1658, Sgt. Major Lambert Closse, one of Maisonneuve's soldiers, was given a grant of 100 arpents in this neighbourhood. He built his house on what is now the corner of St. Dominique and Dorchester Streets, and fortified it against Indian attacks, in one of which he eventually was killed. (Les Contes de la Société Saint-Jean Baptiste de Montréal: No. 14. E. Z. Massicotte.)

burgh men. P. Loedel, a naval surgeon, joined the staff a little later. He died of typhus fever, and the tablet to him is the oldest memorial in the hospital. A very fair idea of the life of the hospital may be gained from its various records, of its personnel, the meals, the patients, the equipment, etc.

We are told:

> "The wages of all female servants shall be not more than $5.00 per month, and of the man servant not more than $8.00 per month.
>
> Their diet shall be tea and bread and butter for breakfast and supper, meat and soup for dinner, and 7 gallons of beer a week. Butter not to exceed 6 lbs. per week. The matron to be allowed 2 lbs. per week." Later on they were also given 3 ozs. of tea per week each, and 1 lb. of Muscovada sugar.

The allowance of beer, however, was subject to change. On September 18, 1833, the Committee ordered that the night nurse be given no more beer, but receive tea instead.

For a long time (up to 1850) the hospital kept its own cows for its milk supply. As early as 1825 there is mention of two cows being bought, with corresponding supplies of hay, because the milkman who had formerly supplied the hospital had given up. The price paid for milk then was about five cents a quart, winter price, and four cents, summer. In 1847 two more cows were bought, to be returned if they were not good milkers. One of them had to be exchanged, as being "too delicate in her feed". But in 1850 the cows evidently proved insufficient and tenders for milk supplies were called for, the price arranged for being even less than four cents per quart.

The staff of the hospital for the first ten years was very small. A matron, Mrs. Stevenson, two nurses and a house surgeon, Dr. Lyons, who was also apothecary, an orderly and a cook, made up the number. Domestic differences occasionally arose, as for instance when the inspecting governors reported:

> "Observing some marks of improper conduct on the face of the cook, we inquired the cause of it from Mrs. Stevenson, to which she replied that the servant man, Joshua, had beaten her."

The matron on this occasion evidently took full advantage of the luxury of being asked to speak, and told the committee of many

3

other things, not only about the cook but also about one of the nurses, a Mrs. Flynn. In the case of the latter, however, she caught a tartar, as in the inquiry which came about Mrs. Flynn retorted with the most circumstantial details of the matron's entertaining friends on food meant for the patients, and so on. Nothing happened, however, except that the cook and Joshua both lost their places.

Then later on, in 1848, Dr. G. E. Fenwick, acting as apothecary, insisted on keeping a dog in his room "to the great annoyance of the servants". He was asked to put it away, but would not, and the Committee of Management had to deal with the matter. It was decided to take away his privilege of a separate table for his meals, and to make him dine with the steward and matron.[1] But Fenwick forestalled his punishment by resigning. Later on he became one of the chief surgeons of the hospital. He is described as having a charming personality, but he had no idea of time, and was called "the late Dr. Fenwick".

II

For the first sixty years and more there was nothing at all corresponding to our modern ideas of nursing. Even the matrons were little more than magnified housekeepers. The first matron, Mrs. Stevenson, was appointed with the proviso *ad vitam aut ad culpam*, at a salary of £30 per year; a wage which might not drive her "*ad culpam*", but would hardly tempt her to remain "*ad vitam*". However, she proved to be an excellent servant to the institution. She died of cholera contracted on duty.

In the first 15 years there were seven matrons. Mrs. Stevenson; Mrs. Bland and Mrs. Jackson died of typhus fever; another, unnamed, was discharged; Mrs. Griffin died of "fever"; Mrs. Gillis was discharged, and Mrs. Ball was replaced.

Those who actually nursed the patients were quite untrained. They were engaged by the month, and the chief requirement seems

---

[1] Originally, they all dined together. In 1834 the steward and apothecary complained that the matron insisted on keeping a separate table, "contrary to the express instructions of the Committee, and serving them after she had helped herself. The matron, heard in reply, admitted the two tables, but ascribed it to the steward being unpleasant."

to have been that they should be married women; at any rate, those mentioned were usually married. In one instance it is recorded that the cook was made nurse instead of one who was "incompetent". Quite frequently they were chosen from amongst those who had been patients in the wards, as is shown in the following extract from the minutes of the Committee of Management, June 29, 1861:

> "The matron reported that Mrs. Laffoley had given notice of her intention to leave her situation, and that she had engaged Mrs. Wilkins, a patient in the hospital, to replace her at the rate of $6.00 per month. Mrs. Inglis, at present a patient in the hospital, has been placed in charge of Ward 24, at the rate of $5.00 per month."

Many of these women, however, must have had a natural instinct for nursing, and too, there must have been some whose experience and natural sagacity was of great value in the hospital. This was so in the case of St. Bartholomew's in London. An instance is quoted in the history of that institution of one such wise old nurse actually showing an erring house surgeon when and how to compress the posterior tibial artery.[1] As will be seen later on in the history of our hospital, the time came when the medical men were glad to turn to the histories kept by the nurses. Apparently, for many years, very scanty records of the patients were kept, there being little beyond their name and diagnosis.

We have no detailed accounts of the medical treatment, but can gather a good deal about it indirectly. The methods were probably as good as could be found anywhere else. The hospital carried on teaching of medical students from its earliest years, and that tended to keep up the standard of treatment. In accordance with the views of the day bleeding was a frequent practice. Orders for bleeding basins are found in the records. Drugs, of course, occupied a much larger place in treatment than nowadays, and prescription books as far back as 1845 have been preserved. Alcoholic stimulants were a routine. Whisky would be ordered by the 10-gallon lot, even in the hospital's first year, and the Committee of Management frequently discussed the supply of liquor needed. Sometimes it is recorded that they sampled the brandy and port wine before ordering hogsheads of them.

---

[1] *History of St. Bartholomew's Hospital:* Sir Norman Moore.

The taking of temperatures, of course, could not have been done much before the "seventies". The pocket thermometer was only perfected in 1868, by Clifford Allbutt. The early records frequently mention orders for "thermometers" but these must have been for watching the room temperature in the wards.

Amongst minor details may be mentioned the early recommendation that a "Sedan chair be procured for the purpose of transporting patients from their respective wards to and from the Baths." Nightcaps for the patients were part of the wardrobe; they appear early in the list of hospital stores. One other unusual item amongst the early purchases of the hospital is that of "twelve spittoons". These were evidently meant for the wards; at one point a complaint appears regarding their misuse by the patients. It may be added that the patients were evidently more unruly than in the present day, as the quarterly reports repeatedly show discharges for "irregular conduct". One of the common offences was smoking. One entry in the Governors' Visiting Book is as follows:

"We find that some of the Patients lately, in violation of the rules, smoaked occasionally; we did what we thought necessary to counteract this dangerous propensity, but we make this note more to put the governors that may succeed us on their guard, so that they may also continue their endeavours to put down this evil immediately, as some of the Patients to avoid detection, have been known to hide their pipes hastily in their straw beds, to the great danger of the building."

The matter is referred to again as follows:

"The means of preserving a light during the night in the wards is not as certain or as safe as it should be. The present mode of burning a floating light of oil in a tumbler is attended with many inconveniences, the patients get at it during the night, move it about and often put it out, and it is feared attempt to light pipes and segars at it."

The danger of fire in the building must have been an ever-present one, and the complete absence of any fire escapes until very much later in the history of the hospital, must have been a great source of anxiety. The lighting was done by lamps and lanterns until 1841, when there was a proposal to introduce gas, "provided the Committee of Management be satisfied of the decided economy of the change, and the medical board do approve of it."

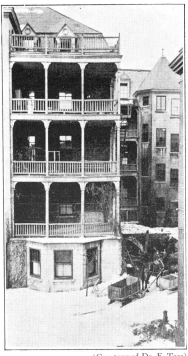

SHOWING THE OLD MORLAND
WING FROM BEHIND, LATER CON-
VERTED TO MEDICAL WARDS.

Towards the right, under the centre
building, can be seen the arch of the
old bricked-in cesspool which was un-
covered in building operations.

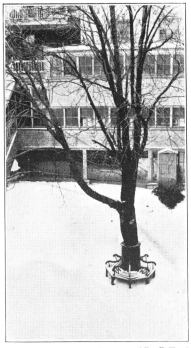

TREE IN OLD GARDEN BEHIND
THE HOSPITAL.

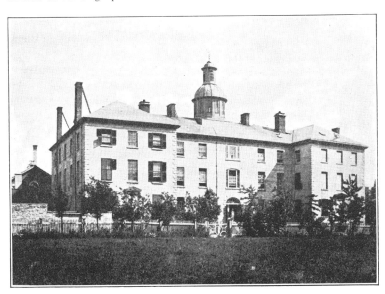

THE HOSPITAL AS ORIGINALLY PLANNED, FINISHED IN 1848 BY
THE ADDITION OF THE REID WING.

III

The hospital played a large part in the great epidemics of cholera, typhus and smallpox which form such striking episodes in the medical history of Montreal. The great cholera year was 1832-33, and the chief typhus epidemic in 1847. In that year the hospital erected sheds and tents to take care of the excess numbers of typhus patients, and the strain on the nursing and medical services was extremely heavy. Dr. Caldwell and Dr. Blackwood (who had served at the "House of Recovery") both died of typhus, as did also two matrons, Mrs. Bland and Mrs. Jackson, and several servants in the institution.

The admission books again give very interesting sidelights on the types of disease in the hospital. Fevers outnumbered all others. There is no doubt about there having been typhus, but probably many cases of typhoid were included under that diagnosis at first. The diagnosis "synochus" was used for a fever which could not be classified; it was a very frequent diagnosis. Another term of great elasticity was "psora". This referred to skin conditions which could not be made to fit into a more definite description. We have exchanged it for "eczema"! Some other terms not now used were, "gelatio", which was common in certain years; "white-swelling" (tuberculosis of the knee joint), "noli me tangere" (rodent ulcer); "porrigo furfurans" (an eczema of the scalp); "emansio mensium" (failure of menses to become established) "dolor capitis" (headache).

The nurses themselves are seldom mentioned; a reference to them by Sir William Osler is well worth recording.[1]

"When I entered the Montreal General Hospital, where I began the study of medicine in 1868, we had the old time nurses. They were generally ward servants who had evolved from the kitchen or from the backstairs into the wards. Many of them were devoted women, many of them became very well trained nurses, but not all of them. Many of them were of the old type so well described by Dickens, and there are some of the senior medical men present who remember the

[1] From an "Address" by Sir Wm. Osler to the Nurses' Training School, Johns Hopkins, Johns Hopkins Nurses' Alumnae Magazine, July 1913, vol. 12, p. 72. Dr. W. W. Francis, librarian of the Osler Library, kindly drew this to my attention.

misery that was necessary in connection with that old-fashioned type of nurse.

Very often, of course, we medical students had to take part in the nursing. In every serious case it was generally the privilege and the duty of the clinical clerk or the surgical dresser to sit up with his patient and attend to the night nursing, as there was only one night nurse to two or three wards. However, there were among these women very remarkable instances of intelligence and devotion. I passed through two or three of the severe epidemics of smallpox in Montreal, and the memory of two of those nurses stands out with great clearness and is today very precious to me. One, a Miss Lancashire, was in looks the old-fashioned Dickensian nurse, but in behaviour, in devotion and in capability equal to the best I have ever met. She nursed smallpox with a rare combination of devotion and skill, and it is always a pleasure to me to look back on those days in which I was associated with her.

The other was a very different type of woman, one of the sisters of a French order of nursing. She was a high-bred woman, who had left her own country and had devoted her life to the work of charity. She had a remarkable career in Montreal, as she had charge of the large civic smallpox hospital. Though I was not formally associated with her, yet she, knowing I was interested in special aspects of the disease, invariably sent a carriage for me when certain cases came in. Interested as I was in the study of the morbid activity of the more malignant types—the terrible black smallpox— I have seen an extraordinary number of the more virulent forms of the disease with her. She herself was often the only person I could get to assist me in the work."

We also have a typically forcible description of the early nursing from the late Dr. F. J. Shepherd, but due allowance must be made for the natural vigour of his style:

"In my day (the late 'sixties and after) age and frowsiness seemed the chief attributes of the nurse, who was ill-educated and was often made more unattractive by the vinous odour of her breath. Cleanliness was not a feature either of the nurse, the ward or the patient; each one did as best pleased her, and her 'langwidge' was 'frequent and painful and free'.

If the day nurse was bad, the night nurse was worse, and as a solatium to help her to bear the burthen of the night, the stimulants which were then freely prescribed for patients to make up perhaps for the lessened tone due to purging and sepsis, often found their way down her throat. One nurse had charge of several wards on different flats, and if a patient was violent, or even delirious, he was strapped down to his bed. I remember on one occasion having operated on a man for strangulated hernia, and there being no one to restrain him, the patient got out of bed and sat on the back gallery, then he helped himself to tap water and drank milk which was at the bedside of other patients, and also ate bread. I found this out accidentally from another patient and complained about it, so next night when I went down I found my patient gagged and strapped hand and foot to the bed to prevent him from misbehaving again. The man got a pneumonia of which he died.

Armies of rats frequently disported themselves about the wards and picked up stray scraps left by the patients, and sometimes attacked the patients themselves."

CHAPTER II

We know something of the working conditions of the nurses in the early days from the Hospital House Rules for 1861:

"OF THE MATRON

"The Matron shall visit the wards of the hospital every morning at eight, every afternoon at one, and every evening at eight o'clock, and oftener if necessary; at these visits she shall see that the wards are properly attended by the nurses, and that all the patients are in their respective wards, and report to the house-surgeon the names of such patients as are absent without leave from their respective wards.

She shall oversee the conduct of the patients and servants. and take care that the wards, apartments, beds, clothes, linen, etc., are kept clean and in good order.

She shall prevent anything being taken into wards except that which is ordered.

She shall not absent herself from the Hospital without the knowledge of the House-Surgeon.

OF THE NURSES

When a patient is admitted into the Hospital, it shall be the duty of the nurse to whose ward such patient may be ordered to see that he or she receives a thorough bath, unless a special order to the contrary be given in writing, by the admitting Medical Officer. She shall give him or her a Hospital shirt and night-cap, and shall deliver without delay, his or her clothes, after an inventory of them has been taken, to the person ordered by the Steward to receive them.

They shall be in their respective wards at 6½ o'clock a.m., each morning, and have them clean and in proper order by 9 a.m.

The Nurses shall be diligent in complying with the orders of the Medical Officers, Surgeon and Matron, and they shall behave with tenderness to the patients.

They shall pay particular attention to the patients, and as often as necessary supply them with the drink prescribed, and assist them when they are unable to assist themselves, and when they are able shall place the vessel or vessels containing their drink commodiously within their reach, and take care that they never remain empty."

It is to be remembered that if the nursing was crude, the payment for it was at the lowest possible rate, as has been said. The wages of the nurses were no better than those of the hospital servants. In the monthly expense lists there are entries of the salary paid the matron, but nothing referring to the nurses as such. They were included under "servants".

In 1859 we find the Committee of Management discussing the rate of wages for the nurses, and it was agreed "to postpone the matter till next week for further consideration". But it was five months before the subject was again taken up. In May 1860 the minute reads:

> "It was agreed that all nurses should be allowed for the future $6.00 per month, at the discretion of the matron, and it is to be understood that ordinary or inferior nurses will remain at $5.00 per month. The kitchen maid (assistant cook) to receive for the future $5.00 per month at the discretion of the matron in place of $4.00."

In 1863 the matter comes up again:

> "The repeated changes in the nurses in the Hospital having been brought to the notice of the Committee, it is deemed expedient to raise the wages of such as retained their situations over one year to $7.00 per month."

There is plenty of proof of these "repeated changes". On November 9, 1855, for example, we read:

> "The matron reported having discharged Mrs. Baker, nurse in the gentlemen's wards, for drunkenness."

and on Feb. 1, 1856:

> "The matron reported night nurse Mrs. Stewart having behaved with such immorality she was obliged to discharge her immediately, and also C. Sawler, outside orderly, on the same account, and also a housemaid of the name of A. Francis for her temper. Also that Margaret Watson, day nurse, and Mrs. Crawford, day nurse, were discharged, the first for bad conduct, and the latter for incapacity."

On another occasion Nov. 19, 1864:

> "The matron was instructed to give the usual notice of dismissal to Mrs. McHaney, the night nurse, in consequence of her having been in a state of inebriety."

11

Some idea of the management of the wards may be gained from the following incident:

> "The matron reported that a Mrs. Pike,([1]) lately matron in the House of Refuge, having made a request to sit up with a patient of the name of Harriet Tanner, who died early on the morning of Sunday, April 18th, such permission was granted. That shortly after H. Tanner's decease Mrs. Pike left the hospital, carrying with her a basket, six shillings and tenpence, a gold ring, and other small matters—deceased property—and the property had been recovered."

Again, on December 5, 1856:

> "Jas. Patton declared to the president that whilst he was in the hospital he had seen the orderly give to a patient of the name of Cavanagh several pints of milk extra; to add thereto he gave him mutton chops and other things. Besides also there was a regular custom of smoking in the ward he was in after three o'clock in the morning."

There is proof, however, that the hospital authorities made the best of the material they had to work with. They showed due appreciation of faithful work, whilst never omitting to inculcate thrift. There was the case of Elizabeth Hoskins, one of the maids, who after having worked as un unpaid servant of all work for nearly five years, was granted $3.00 per month, this "to be deposited in the savings bank in the name of the chairman of the Committee of Management".

This was on October 9, 1869. Poor Elizabeth did not enjoy her affluence very long. On April 1, 1871, the record shows "Elizabeth Hoskins, the old housemaid, died in the institution March 27, 1871. We thus desire to acknowledge the loss of a faithful servant to the hospital, yet to bow with submission to the all wise dispensation of Him who doeth all things well".

But even this did not quite close the story. A little later on we read in the Committee of Management minutes: "Eliz. Hoskins having left $36.00 in the bank, but fearing lest that this should be wasted if given to her friends, it was suggested that the steward

---

([1]) Evidently this Mrs. Pike was serving in the capacity of a "watcher". This was a recognized occupation in the London hospitals early in the 19th century. Women were brought in for the night to watch at the bedside of dying patients.

arrange with them to put a headstone on her grave". The friends
wanted the money, however, for the next and last entry reads:

> "Regarding the Hoskin family, the steward to arrange
> the matter amicably, and authority granted to the treasurer
> to draw the money."

Again, in 1872 (May 18)

> "It being reported that the nurse Charlotte Darley,
> who has been in the service of the hospital 14 years, was
> about to be married, it was agreed to purchase for her a
> sideboard of the value of $30.00, as a testimony of the sense
> entertained by the Committee of her long and faithful
> services."

And on September 23, 1872, Mrs. Wright, who had been night
nurse for eleven years, on her resignation, was voted $25.00 as a
gratuity in consideration of her valuable services.

Matrons came and went fairly quickly. Sometimes married
couples served as steward and matron. A Mr. and Mrs. Symmers
in 1855 wanted to bring their two daughters with them and this
was agreed to, their board to be at the rate of £25 per annum.([1])
"It would be better to allow her to come in," said the Committee,
"as it would encourage her in the performance of her duties."

Six years later another matron is recorded as having two
daughters living in the hospital, but by now the rate of board had
been raised to £35 per annum. At the same time the Board considered the case of Dr. Taylor, the house surgeon, who announced
that he was going to get married, and wanted to have his wife
boarding with him in the hospital. This was agreed to, the charge
being $80.00 per month including washing, and taking their meals
with the other officers of the institution.

In 1866 (April 11) the Committee of Management records
for the first time signs of trying to raise the standard of nursing,

> "The matron was requested to make arrangements as
> follows: to engage a better class of nurses than those at present
> in the hospital, giving them an advance on the wages now
> paid, their duty to be to attend to the patients. Also, to

([1]) One of these daughters later established her well-known school for girls
in Montreal. The other became the wife of Dr. R. Craik, who was Dean
of the Medical Faculty of McGill University.

engage charwomen to do the cleaning of the windows, washing of dishes, and otherwise all the work now done by the nurses, except the attendance on patients.

The nurses' wages to be as follows: $7.00 per month for the first year, with a bonus of $12.00 at the end of the year if found worthy of it."

What may have resulted from this is not recorded, but it was six years before the subject is mentioned again. This time the Committee instructs the matron (March 16, 1872) "to procure such nurses as she deems best, and what may be necessary to tend to the comfort of the patients, whether these be in the fever or the general hospital."

II

By the time the hospital reached its fiftieth year it began to be realized by the management that the buildings were becoming inadequate, both from the point of view of age and on account of the growing numbers of patients. After the addition of the Richardson and Reid wings there was little change beyond the very important acquisition in 1866 of the land opposite the hospital, on which the nurses' home now stands. This gave much needed open space. In 1867 an infectious diseases hospital with forty beds was added, in the rear of the Richardson wing. Smallpox was for long years an accepted visitation in the city and this building was in use until 1885, when the overwhelming epidemic of the disease caused the civic authorities to open their own isolation hospital and relieve the strain. It was not until 1893, however, that infectious diseases were finally separated from the hospital admissions.

William Osler was in charge of the smallpox building in 1875, and himself contracted the disease, though in a mild form. It was finally turned into a laundry and then pulled down to make room for the new wing.

Another addition was made in 1874, in the form of a children's ward, which was behind the Reid wing. This was called the Morland wing, in memory of Mr. Thos. Morland, who was an outstanding benefactor of the hospital. This wing was afterwards used for medical wards.

There were no other additions until 1892, which will be referred to later. But in 1877 the introduction of Lister's antiseptic methods by Dr. T. G. Roddick caused a revolution in hospital methods. Surgical work increased tremendously and the demands on the hospital became much heavier. It was realized that the building was inadequate in many ways, but the management did not feel that they could provide for the very large expenditures necessary for new buildings. There are frequent reports by those making the weekly inspections to show how much improvements were needed.

For example, on July 26, 1871, Mr. E. W. A. Prentice suggests

> "that the rule regarding the change of bed linen once a week should be relaxed where necessary; for example, a boy with an abscess in his leg should have his sheets changed much oftener."

And on September 30, 1871,

> "We noticed in the matter of bed linen that things were tolerably well worn." (Messrs. John J. Arnton and Chas. Binmore.)

On August 3, 1871, Mr. Prentice again reports:

> "I visited the wards and found many of the patients suffering great annoyance from the number of flies, and beg leave most respectfully to suggest that the ordinary means be taken to investigate this evil."

No one subject received more attention than the ventilation of the building. Sometimes it was merely referred to as being defective, but now and then specific sources are mentioned. For example, the "deadhouse" was close up under the windows of the wards, and many times it was recommended by visiting governors that it should be moved somewhere else. Mr. Geo. McRae alone made the recommendation twice: "It is," he said, "exposed to the view of the patients in some of the wards, and in other respects may be unpleasant owing to the effluvia which must escape from it."

Garbage tins were left under the windows, and were complained about. Rats were mentioned. Mr. H. Archibald on July 11, 1873, reported:

> "I note that the house is badly infested with rats, and would respectfully suggest that something surely can be done

to abate this terrible nuisance, which would not be tolerated in any private house."

On March 19, 1875, Mr. John Crawford remarks:

"One of the wards, however, has a very disagreeable odour, proceeding apparently from an advanced consumptive patient."

Two years later he makes the mild suggestion that

"if not interfering with the patients I would suggest the admission of a little fresh air into the halls."

On November 9th, 1885, Messrs. Strachan Bethune and C. Lane reported that things were clean and apparently well ventilated, and added, rather gratuitously perhaps, that "they failed to detect any bad odours". Some humourist has pencilled in the margin of the report; "! ! ! ! Try again. Better luck next time".

Incidentally, one report, having dealt faithfully with the ventilation and many other things, including the shortcomings of the other governors, turned to another subject mentioned by no one else at any time:

"We would beg leave to suggest as an improvement the reduction of the quantity of intoxicating drinks in present use in the Montreal General Hospital, for the following reason; that many patients, when convalescent or discharged having acquired a liking for the use of stimulants, will be inclined to want it." (George Rogers and H. Mills.)

But there is never anything but praise in these reports for the way in which the patients were nursed and treated.

CHAPTER III

In 1874 comes the first suggestion of the formation of a training school for nurses. At this time the matron was a Miss Forbes, a lady of good family from St. Andrews.

"Committee of Management, February 23, 1874. Resolved that it is expedient that a system of trained hospital nurses, such as approved of in England, should be introduced into the hospital. That this committee apply to the governors for the necessary authority to introduce such a system, and procure trained nurses with the support of the hospital, or otherwise as the committee may deem expedient."

On November 11th, the scheme is again referred to and recommended. At this time also the need for enlarging the hospital was brought up.

The report to the governors on the matter is as follows:

"The Committee of Management have had under anxious consideration the desirability of procuring a staff of trained nurses for the hospital. They feel that while the step is essential to the due efficiency of the institution, it would entail additional expense; but they cannot for a moment doubt that it is the duty of the governors to make the hospital thoroughly efficient, and adopt all available means tending to promote the speedy recovery of the patients.

The training of nurses by the institution would be of great public benefit, and would give the hospital a large additional claim on the community. The committee have entered into correspondence with a lady in England, and have good hopes of being able to make a satisfactory arrangement, if the governors give their sanction to the undertaking."

Then there was some correspondence (which was not kept) with Miss Maria Machin, of St. Thomas's Hospital, London,([1]) with a view to securing her services as lady superintendent, together with some trained nurses. Miss Machin eventually came out in September, 1875, bringing one trained nurse with her. Three others followed a little later. Evidently they had to put up with some

---

([1]) Probably Miss Nightingale was approached at first, but the minutes refer only to correspondence with Miss Machin.

inconvenience at first, as a note in the minutes reads (September 27, 1875): "It was agreed to appropriate the room formerly occupied by the steward as bedroom and office as the nurses' dining room, there being no accommodation of that kind at present; suitable furniture to be provided."

Miss Machin entered upon her duties on Saturday, October 2, 1875.

This development originated when Mr. William Molson was president, Mr. Charles Alexander, vice-president, and Dr. R. P. Howard, secretary.

Further efforts were now made to develop the training of nurses. In May, 1876, the Committee of Management authorized the lady superintendent,

> "to engage in England four competent trained nurses, one of whom shall be a ward sister. The hospital will pay passages out to Montreal. The salary of the ward sister shall be £40, £45 and £50 for the three years. The wages of the sisters shall be £30, £35 and £40. The ward sister shall, as part of her duties, assist in the training of nurses and the other nurses engaged shall also render all the assistance in their power in the same duty."

On July 31, 1876, four more nurses arrived from St. Thomas's (one of the original four, Miss Martha Rice, had died of typhoid not long after her arrival), and it was specifically arranged that they were to train probationers.

A note in the minutes on October 2, 1876, shows that the conditions in the hospital were causing comment, as a letter was read before the committee from Miss Machin, enclosing letters from Mr. Bonham Carter and Miss Nightingale about the sanitary conditions in the hospital. The letters, however, do not seem to have been kept.([1])

([1]) There is reason to believe that Miss Machin had written to Miss Night-ingale about the hospital conditions, as there are letters from the latter to Miss Machin which are preserved in London. Unfortunately, they are not readily available.

At any rate, it is likely that the hospital was inspected officially at this time. An entry in the Governors' Visiting Book made on Sept. 14, 1897 (the year in which the foundation stone of the Nurses' Home was laid), reads as follows:

"Through the kindness of Mr. Wolferstan Thomas and Mr. Ewing we have thoroughly gone over the hospital and are charmed with every-thing, the contrast since we visited it many years ago being most wonder-ful . . . (Signed) R. A. A. Jones, Mary E. Lynn, Caroline M. Arnott, of London, England."

Evidently some of the English nurses found other positions, as on July 30, 1877, Miss Machin reports the expected arrival of two more nurses from the Nightingale Training School to replace two (Masters and Marsh) who were leaving. Incidentally, the bringing over of these two new nurses had not been arranged through the Committee, and they were "surprised" and wanted an explanation from the President.

II

Under date of September 26, 1877, there is a very comprehensive report from a special committee, on the cost of running the hospital. It lays great emphasis on the value of the nurses from England, but criticises the number of servants, giving details of the management which are interesting.

"There are at present 30 nurses and assistants. In large hospitals elsewhere one attendant to every six patients is considered a very full staff. As the average number of patients in the hospital is less than 140, the staff of nurses ought to be very carefully considered.

The trained nurses brought from England have been of very great service and the retention of a certain number of these is most desirable. They should take the lead in various wards, and be able accordingly to train up nurses in this country, whose services would prove of very great advantage in future, and by degrees secure a well trained and efficient staff of nurses.

The other female servants employed, consisting of cooks, housemaids, laundry women, etc., should be carefully looked after to check extravagance and waste. There are at present ten employed on these duties. There is also a man cook."

Then come some remarks which show that the idea of the training school was losing ground:

"In the opinion of the undersigned the proper plan of supervision would be to obtain the services of a matron of the best experience that can be obtained, who should be placed over the various nurses and women servants, who should be responsible for the proper cleanliness of the hospital, the efficient discharge of their duties by the women servants, the proper care of the linen, etc., and the economical and proper use of the food required in the hospital.

It is not necessary to have anyone in charge but an experienced matron such as here spoken of, who will give her personal, hourly attention to the duties to be laid down by the Committee of Management.

The undersigned must now refer to the lady superintendent, who has been connected with the hospital for the last two years, and whose term of engagement is about expiring. One of the main objects contemplated when Miss Machin joined the hospital was the establishment of a training school for nurses. This it has been found impossible to put in force. It would appear, therefore, undesirable to make any renewed engagement with Miss Machin, as in the absence of any training school the management of the hospital can be made more effective and economical by the mode already recommended.

That the system of nursing has been greatly improved during the time that the trained nurses have been employed is beyond doubt, and your committee are glad to recognize the fitness of Miss Machin to carry on such training school as was proposed, but as that is now impracticable it is necessary that the management of the hospital in future should be conducted solely on the footing which the funds at our disposal render not only desirable but imperative.

(Signed) Chas. Alexander,
John Plimsoll,
F. H. Bryson."

Apparently, Miss Machin did not see things in the same light. She was called before the Committee and a long interview was held, which, however, as the record states "in its results failed to satisfy the Committee." This led to the resolution:

"That the request made to the Lady Superintendent to suggest any means of economy having failed after a full interview with her to produce any response which promises any material reduction, the committee must deal with the whole question in the manner which best commends itself to their judgment.

That the cost of conducting the hospital now exceeds by at least $10,000 a year the funds available, and it is therefore recommended that the number of nurses be reduced from 25 to not exceeding 20.

That a matron shall be appointed who shall reside permanently in the hospital; have control of all the nurses and women servants, supervise cooking in the kitchen, and see that there is no waste or extravagance; be held responsible for the hospital being kept in a proper state of cleanliness, and control the washing and proper care of the laundry.

That convalescent patients be employed to aid the regular servants, when the house surgeon considers them fit to do so, in order that the number of servants to be paid by the hospital may be kept within the smallest numbers.

That the proposal to establish a training school for nurses having for financial necessity fallen through, the hospital can no longer afford the expenses of a lady superintendent, and the committee must therefore with regret consider the necessity forced upon them to part with Miss Machin, now that the term of her engagement is about expiring.

In coming to this determination in view of the present financial position and requirements of the hospital the committee desire to take the opportunity of expressing their full appreciation of the great interest which Miss Machin has exhibited in the care of the patients, and her excellent qualities in everything that relates to the important question of nursing. In parting with her the committee will be glad most carefully to consider the fair and proper consideration which is due to her and desire to make the severance as regards time upon the most proper and liberal basis."

A special meeting of the Committee of Management was held on September 28, 1877, to consider this report. At first an attempt was made to disregard the recommendations referring to Miss Machin. But the motion to this effect was lost (proposed by Mr. Lunn, seconded by Mr. Gault). Then it was decided to see if the English nurses could be induced to remain.

This all went to the Medical Board, who replied *inter alia:*

"That with reference to the suggestion of the sub-committee that considerable reduction in the number of servants might be made, this Board would desire to express its decided opinion (founded mainly upon the statements of the present attending physicians) that the staff of actual nurses, i.e., those in immediate attendance upon patients, is by no means in excess of what is really required to ensure a degree of proper care in this all important work. On enquiry, the Board are informed that the number of nurses employed at the present time is as follows:

Head day nurses 6; assistants 9; night nurses 6; making 15 nurses actually on duty in the daytime, or an average of $9\frac{1}{3}$ patients per nurse. In addition to the nurses, 7 women are employed in the wards for the purpose of keeping them clean, and in other ways assisting the nurses, and were not such assistance given we are of the opinion that the 15 nurses would not be sufficient for the proper nursing of the patients."

As regards the replacement of the lady superintendent by a matron, the Medical Board had this to say:

"The Medical Board desire respectfully to dissent from their recommendation. In the treatment of all disease, good nursing is of the utmost importance, and without this, medical advice would be powerless for good. In order to have nursing properly performed it is highly advisable that the nurses should be under the control of a lady capable of instructing them in their duties and consequently commanding their respect.

The Board therefore would strongly deprecate any action which would have the effect of substituting a non-trained matron for a skilled lady superintendent.

On October 6, 1877, the Medical Board passed the following resolution:

"Moved by Dr. Reddy and seconded by Dr. Ross, that whereas this Board have learned that the present lady superintendent is about to sever her connection with the hospital: Resolved that the members of this Board hereby record their sense of the careful, kind and efficient manner in which Miss Machin has invariably performed her important duties in connection with the nursing department of the hospital; and beg to express their high appreciation of the beneficial changes in the system and efficiency of the nursing that have been carried out during Miss Machin's term of office.

They regret that circumstances of a pecuniary nature should have arisen to oblige the committee to dispense with the valuable services of Miss Machin."

III

The following letter from Miss Machin to the Committee of Management is worthy of record:

"The recent action of the Committee of Management with regard to myself, and the consequent public discussion of the domestic affairs of the institution in the newspapers and otherwise, have given me great pain. I do not now write for the purpose of justifying any part of the administration of my department, but as much of the trouble seems to have arisen from an erroneous impression that I had declined to carry

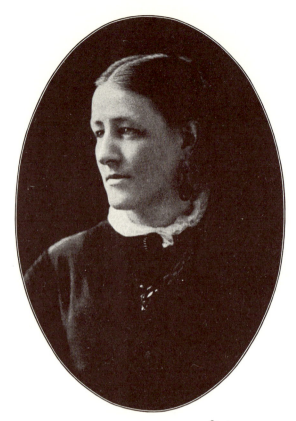

MISS MARIA MACHIN IN 1875.

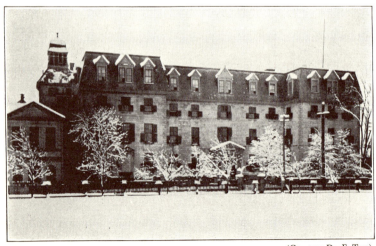

SHOWING THE OLD PATHOLOGICAL BUILDING IN FRONT, AND THE
SMALLPOX HOSPITAL WITH ITS TOWER BEHIND.

out the orders of the Committee, I desire to say to you that I am not aware of having done so in any instance.

I fully appreciate the manner in which I have been until lately sustained by the Committee, and nothing could be further from my wishes than any want of harmony between us.

The welfare of the institution is the object we all have in view, and it is my desire to cooperate with the Committee in reducing expenditure wherever that can be done without sacrificing efficiency.

In my opinion, some of the recent recommendations of the Committee would, if carried into effect, be injurious to the hospital and inconsistent with the retention of trained nurses, at any rate from the Nightingale Home.

I should be glad if the Committee would reconsider the recommendations to reduce the number of nurses and female servants. In the present financial condition of the hospital I am aware that every possible reduction should be made, but I do not think that the expectations of the committee can be altogether realized.

I am, Dear Sir
Yours faithfully,
Maria M. Machin."

At the meeting of the Committee of Management on November 14, 1877, it was decided to retain Miss Machin. Various economies were put into force; these included the not taking in of any more infectious cases, and the using of their ward for general cases; the closing of two wards; the getting rid of the night door-keeper, his duties to be attended to by the nurse nearest the door; the dispensing with the services of seven nurses. It is on record that the Committee never had any intention of dispensing with the services of the nurses from England.

It was also made clear that Miss Machin's appointment was *not* for a limited period, and that it was contingent upon her establishing a school for nurses.

The following description from a newspaper article of the time (1877) gives an idea of the inadequacy of the hospital.

"There is only one bathroom for all the wards on the male side of the hospital. It is most inconveniently located and, in short, is entirely inadequate for the purposes for which it was designed. The water-closets are in its immediate vicinity and, as if some malevolent genius of unfitness had taken charge of the arrangements, the shaft by which the meals are hoisted from the lower regions is only separated from both by a wooden partition. Meals are prepared for distribution on the landing in full sight of this trinity of incompatibilities."

Then comes a catalogue of deficiencies:

"The smallness of the wards, allowing an insufficiency of cubic inches to each bed; the poverty of window room; the scanty means for natural, and the absurd attempts at artificial ventilation throughout a large proportion of the wards, and the total absence of anything that deserves the name of light in some of the passages; the impossibility of admitting many essential conveniences from want of space; the unavoidably unwholesome condition of the walls from age and porosity of material, allowing them to become impregnated with various miasmata; the shocking accommodation for violent weak-minded patients in the basement, more like provocatives to insanity than prophylactic agencies; the situation of laundry immediately under the wards, aggravated by the ease with which noxious vapours therefrom can ascend to the first flat, imparting in their passage quaint, unwelcome flavours to flesh, fish and fowl; the wholly uncalled-for little nests of pestilence which obtrude themselves with disagreeable familiarity at almost every turn and corner in this Tartarean No-man's-land; may be included in the bill of objections which we would bring against our otherwise admirable Montreal General Hospital."

IV

The winter went past, but evidently the situation became too difficult, and on May 6, 1878, the quarterly report announced the resignation of Miss Machin, and also, as a consequence, the resignation of Miss Blower and the four English nurses remaining in the hospital. The resignation was accepted with regret, to take effect on June 30th. There is nothing in the records to show what precipitated this.

The Committee recorded the following:

"The standard of nursing in this hospital has been greatly raised since the advent of Miss Machin, and it is desirable in every way that the present standard of nursing should be fully maintained. To this end, the Committee are of the opinion that it will be necessary to make some arrangements for training nurses in the hospital . . .

The Committee are of the opinion that the expenses hitherto incurred in bringing nurses from England have been abundantly compensated for by the beneficial influence of the change upon the whole staff, but nurses cannot be expected to leave their homes unless special inducements are offered. We cannot continue to bring them from England or elsewhere, without permanently raising the scale of wages. There would therefore be a certain degree of economy in training nurses here."

Efforts were made to keep Miss Machin and her nurses, but in the report for the quarter ending July 31, 1878, the Committee has "regretfully to state that the resignations of the foregoing were followed by their leaving the hospital on July 1st".

The Montreal General Hospital was the only instance in which Florence Nightingale nurses were not successful in establishing a training school. That should be taken into account if any judgment is to be passed on this episode in the history of the hospital. Miss Machin must have understood Canadian conditions to some extent, as she had been born in Sherbrooke and was brought up in Quebec City. She was educated in England and then travelled and resided on the Continent for some time, returning to train at St. Thomas's Hospital in London. Miss Nightingale had selected her for the post in Montreal, although according to Miss Livingston, Miss Machin's training had not been complete owing to her having injured her hand. Her career in later life established beyond doubt her qualities of professional leadership.

Miss Machin is described as having an attractive personality, with dignity and force of character, but she was dictatorial and lacking in tact. Apparently she demanded too much of her servants, as the hospital books show a large turnover of these during her short term of office. The wages, of course, were never enough to attract a very good type.

She had the friendship and entire support of some of the members of her Committee, notably Mr. Peter Redpath and Mr. Wm. Robertson, but for some reason or other, she was at variance with some of its other members, such as Mr. Alexander, who, as Miss Livingston puts it was "to say the least, harmless and well meaning."[1] Her position was not made any easier by the loss of

[1] Apparently, Mr. Alexander was extremely zealous in his duties in the hospital. On one of his official tours of inspection he thought he should investigate what was going on behind a screen in one of the wards. Miss Machin came in just as he was looking over the screen and took offense at his well-meaning but not well judged action.

her fiancé, Dr. Jack Cline, a brilliant young member of the staff, who died of diphtheria on September 29, 1877.

The conditions in the hospital must have been enough to test her courage almost to the point of despair, but all accounts agree in praise of her work. The expressions of appreciation from the Committee of Management and Medical Board have already been quoted. The Governors also recorded their admiration, both in formal meeting and through the weekly comments of the visiting governors; for example, on November 24, 1875, Mr. John J. Day, after his round of inspection, says:

> "I found a decided change for the better in many respects, arising evidently out of the interest taken by the new Lady Superintendent, Miss Machin, whom I regard as a great acquisition to the institution."

And Mr. David A. P. Watt, on Sunday, June 30, 1878, says:

> "This being the last day of service from the Lady Super-intendent, Miss Machin, and her staff of trained nurses, the undersigned does here express his regret thereat, and also his conviction that the withdrawal of these ladies from the hospital and from the city is a notable one, and at the present time, a well-nigh irreparable public loss."

V

This rather large gap in the nursing service was filled by secur-ing the return to the hospital of three of the English nurses formerly on the staff. Miss Machin was succeeded by Miss Harriet Rimmer, who without any special training had been interested in hospital work, and was asked by the Committee to take over the super-intendency.

After leaving the hospital Miss Machin and her nurses went to stay for a time with the Gibb family at Como. One of the nurses was a Miss Ellen Webb. The Training School today possesses amongst its archives two small volumes of devotional works which had been presented by Miss Florence Nightingale to Miss Webb, when she came out to Montreal, and they bear inscriptions in Miss Nightingale's writing. Miss Webb's boat was wrecked near the Island of Anticosti on her return to England and she underwent much hardship in a small boat before being rescued by another steamer. One of the books is stained with sea water.

Miss Machin became the Lady Superintendent of St. Bartholomew's in London and held the position from December 12, 1878 to December 8, 1881. Later she married a Mr. Redpath. She went to South Africa and established a hospital at Bloemfontein. Later she was in Kimberley and nursed all through the famous siege of that town in the Boer War. She died in Kimberley, and is buried there.

The following letter from Florence Nightingale to Dr. G. W. Campbell of the hospital, whilst he was on a visit to London, is worthy of reproduction. The original is preserved in the McGill Historical Museum.

April 11/76

AUTOGRAPH LETTER FROM MISS NIGHTINGALE

(Courtesy of *The Canadian Nurse*)

CHAPTER IV

The question of the training school came up again in the following year. The quarterly report for April 30, 1879, contains the expressed hope that before the end of the year it is expected to open a training school under the immediate control of the hospital:

> "The cost of this institution is not likely to be materially felt, and within a very few years the 'Training School' may be partially self-sustaining, provided we can induce the requisite number of young women to enter."

There was evidently some intention of sending out nurses from the hospital, as the report goes on:

> "A considerable revenue will probably be derived from services rendered to private families by nurses who have not completed their time, but who will be quite competent to take charge of a sick room, the charge made by the hospital for such services being in excess of the wages paid to the nurses."

The idea was not developed, however. Nearly a year and a half passed before anything is recorded about it. Then, in 1880 (August 23), the minutes refer to a letter from Miss Rimmer saying that she had been authorized to go to Boston to secure a "Lady Trainer of Nurses". This was Miss Anna Caroline Maxwell, a graduate of the Boston City Hospital

> "the lady who had been recommended as a teacher for our proposed training school. She impressed me favourably (and) all inquiries about her being favourable, I engaged her at a salary of $400.00 per annum."

This was approved, and the president was authorized to ascertain what accommodation could be given in the hospital for the purpose of a training school.

Miss Maxwell arrived in November, 1880. A circular was drawn up, to be sent out around the Townships. It announced that the school would open on January 1, 1881, under a competent lady instructor. Special instruction would also be given by the medical staff. It was intended also to open the school to ladies who might be desirous of joining with remuneration, or who might be willing to pay for the instruction. The course was for two years.

The school did not succeed, although there is little on record to show why. Miss Maxwell resigned in June, 1881. No reasons were given. The committee merely records that they "had pleasure in bearing testimony to her personal character and attainments, and very much regret the severance of her connection with the hospital". No steps were taken to appoint anyone else to run the school, but the committee said they intended that "under the charge of the medical superintendent, instruction in the duties of the nurses would be afforded to all suitable applicants".

Although no reason is given for Miss Maxwell's resignation it is easy to understand why she did not stay when we read her account of conditions in the hospital at the time, written many years later. She had accepted the post at the General soon after her graduation:

"There I found everything bending to the will of the attending staff; hospital funds were taken to purchase champagne to be used in building up the reserve forces of patients to be operated upon, while ragged ticks filled with straw were the only beds provided for the patients, and a basket full of straw could be swept up after the students' rounds.

The laundry was inadequate. Damp linen was sent to the wards to be hung as decorations (?) upon any available space until dry enough to use. The hospital was crowded and there was no division of the services. Available beds were used for surgical or medical cases, as they were admitted, with the result that the lungs of a suffering tuberculous patient were often filled with smoke from his neighbour's pipe, the neighbour being a strong lusty man with a fractured femur.

An attempt had been made to remedy defective ventilation by bringing air into the wards through large pipes a foot in diameter. These pipes were fitted with dampers. The dampers had been closed for years, for pailsful of dust fell when I opened them.

Examination of urine was carried on in the wards. Specimens were placed on a table, and each student examined them at will, from one to two or three days later. Add to this the fact that all lavatory utensils were of opaque china, filled with a sediment of long standing, and you can imagine the resulting odour. After much persuasion, the attending staff

decided to establish a laboratory, and I had one fitted up
in the hospital. When the college opened in the autumn,
however, the request came to return to the old method, as
the student must have the specimen to examine at the bedside
of the patient.

Bedside notes were unknown. In a few instances, I
induced the nurses to keep records of serious cases. Presently
the doctors began to ask to see them, and later, they were
introduced. The surgeons criticised our counting sponges in
cases of abdominal section, but later adopted the method
after several lives had been lost from sponges being left in
the wound.

Plaster casts and bandages were made from one and one-
half to two inches in thickness, with strips of iron on either
side to keep them from breaking, with the result that the
patients were unable to carry them about on leaving their beds.

The nurses were sleeping in cubicles built into an old
ward, and after a stormy night their beds were often festooned
with snow. No sitting-room was provided. The dining room
was presided over by an autocrat who required each nurse to
take her food from a side table, wash her own dishes, and
place them in the cupboard after the meal. There was small
inducement for women of a refined type to enter the school,
only four really suitable candidates offered, and the trustees
decided to defer the plan."[1]

Another account of the hospital at this time appears in a letter
written to the London "*Lancet*" (October 7, 1882). The writer
refers to the hospital as having the appearance of a workhouse.
The wards were spoken of as being clean but the accommodation
everywhere was limited and inconvenient.

"A little chamber, with a few old raised benches is called
the operating room, and does duty also as a chapel.[2] I
presume the operating table covered with a cloth is used for
the communion, the box of sawdust under such a covering
not being visible."

It must also be recorded, however, that in this same year there
appeared in one of the Montreal papers a letter from one who had

---

[1] "*Struggles of the Pioneers*" by Miss Anna C. Maxwell, Presbyterian
Hospital, New York. Read at a meeting of the New York State Nurses'
Association, Albany, New York, October, 1920.

[2] Later on there was a chapel in the pathological building, and later still
this was moved to the present nurses' home. Proper furniture has been
provided for it and services are regularly held in it.

spent some time in the hospital as a patient, extolling the virtues of the institution in the highest terms, mentioning especially the food and the cleanliness.

II

Then came a period without any definite teaching, except for some instruction by the medical staff. However, the class of women taking up nursing was slowly improving. Here is an extract from the report of the medical superintendent, Dr. James Gray, in 1884.

> "The nurses have almost without exception performed their duties satisfactorily. They, as a rule, show themselves to be careful and painstaking in the interests of the hospital. Some of them are very efficient, while others of course are not, simply because they have had no experience in such work; and in this connection I strongly advise that something further be done in the way of training nurses. In my opinion it does not receive half the attention it deserves. In justice to them and in the interest of the institution I think some means should be provided for their training outside of and supplementing their ordinary work."

Outside of the hospital also there was a feeling that a training school should be established. On September 23, 1884, the secretary of the Protestant Associated Charities of Montreal wrote as follows to the Committee of Management:

> "I am desired by the director of the Association to enquire whether it would be practicable to form a nursing class in connection with the hospital, to comprise those who desire to make nursing a vocation, and those who desire to learn nursing for domestic care."

But the Committee of Management had their answer ready:

> "The secretary was instructed to ask Mr. Hollis to define more plainly what was wanted, and where is the money to come from to defray the expenses."

Nothing more was heard from Mr. Hollis.

However, training was kept up as well as possible. Dr. Gray, the superintendent, reports a little later that a class was formed "for the benefit of the nurses, by which means the effort is being made to supplement their ward work". Many applications were received for this class, and several had to be refused. Throughout this period Miss Rimmer's management seems to have been entirely satisfactory. One superintendent, Dr. McClure, makes the comment: "I feel that things are all right when she is around."

After Miss Rimmer had been in charge for some months, the Medical Board were asked by the Committee for their opinion as to making her appointment permanent. The Board recorded that

> "They had much pleasure in testifying to the highly efficient manner in which Miss Rimmer has performed the duties entrusted to her in connection with the hospital. They considered that it would be conducive to the best interests of the institution if her services could be secured in a permanent manner."

Added to this was a recommendation that a trained nurse should be appointed to have general supervision of the other nurses: in effect, a compromise on the plan of a training school.

Miss Rimmer was not a trained nurse. She was an English lady of means, who had come out to Montreal on a visit. She lost her brother under very tragic circumstances and took it very much to heart. From then on she devoted herself to charitable work, and either volunteered or was asked by the Board to act as Lady Superintendent. She brought her own maid, Agnes Murray, who acted as housekeeper, and was probably the individual referred to by Miss Maxwell. Miss Rimmer was stern, but was well liked. She is spoken of as being a good organizer, but her strength did not lie in administration as much as in her character and high ideals. Undoubtedly, she attracted a much better type of woman to take up nursing in the hospital. This was quite evident in the fine qualities of those of her staff who remained to work under Miss Livingston.

CHAPTER V

The conditions in the hospital generally seem to have been very unsatisfactory at this time. Every report contains criticism and complaint. Here for example, is Dr. McClure's report for the quarter ending August 8, 1887:

"Again I beg to call your attention to the inadequacy of the present building, both as regards space and equipment, although the report shows 34 fewer patients treated than during the same quarter last year.

This reduction has taken place in the women's and children's ward, the men's wards having been if possible more overcrowded than last year, notwithstanding the fact that 12 men have been accommodated in the tent ever since the weather became warm enough. I have had as many as eight or ten men sleeping on temporary beds on the floor at night, and have even had to refuse cases that should in the interests of humanity have been admitted.

Again, in these days when success in surgery is found to depend so much on asepsis, it is found impossible to carry out the principle thoroughly owing to the unsanitary condition of the building. The floors are old and worn, in some places actually worn through, forming a nidus for all disease germs. In fact such is the condition of the building that abdominal sections have been abandoned some two years ago or more by nearly all the attending surgeons, when case after case failed that should have succeeded had the building been free from disease infection. This tends to bring discredit not only on the hospital but on the surgeons.

At present there are 35 cases of typhoid in the wards; 22 of these are men. There are only 30 medical beds in the male wards, so that there are only 8 beds for all other medical cases, unless the surgical wards are encroached on.

The want of small wards to isolate noisy, delirious patients is seriously felt. Occasionally there are four or five delirious patients in one ward, making a continual noise, perhaps shouting and annoying their neighbours. In the infectious wing where isolation is attempted there is tolerably good isolation from the main building, but there is practically no isolation of the different diseases from one another, owing

33

to the defective building and the want of nurses. On several occasions patients have come in with one disease, and have taken one or two other diseases before getting out. It is impossible also to prevent vermin, bugs and cockroaches from infesting the cracks in the ward partitions.

The nurses cannot be had because there is no room to accommodate them, their rooms already being overcrowded. Often two beds are put in one room, leaving the occupants hardly room to walk about. These rooms are cold and uncomfortable in winter, and it is impossible to keep them free from bugs in summer. If we had good rooms for the nurses I have no doubt many of the best young women of this country who find their way to American hospitals would stay at home for their training and thus the standard of nursing in this hospital would be raised."

In this year it was decided for the first time to assign a special nurse to the operating room. Miss Alicia Dunne, head of ward 32, was chosen. Incidentally, the operating room was being improved. The medical superintendent reports:

"At present there is no system of artificial light in the operating room, except coal oil lamps. I have received positive instructions not to allow these to be used any longer. It will be necessary to have light in this room, and also more light in the wards. The electric light will be best, on account of the danger of the ether taking fire from a gas jet."

But the Committee of Management were slow to agree. They said, let the same method of lighting continue to be used, "but the oil must be of the finest quality, called luxor oil."

The Superintendent, Kirkpatrick, replied:

"For the operating room coal oil lamps are not sufficient, setting aside the danger from the ether being so near a light. Again, it looks very bad to visitors to have no better form of lighting the operating room of a hospital of this size."

Later on, his report again brings up the matter of the conditions under which the nurses lived.

"On Monday, July 1st, 1889, the nurses appeared in their uniforms for the first time.([1])

More and better accommodation is needed for the nurses. It is getting more and more difficult to fill the vacancies that

---

([1]) These were of a blue wash material.

occur, and soon it will be impossible to get more to come. Some who come refuse to stay unless better rooms are given to them. The rooms are too hot in summer and too cold in winter, and are infested with vermin. The nurses have no place to stay when off duty, nor to receive visitors."

Rats must have been very troublesome also, as at about this time a professional rat-catcher was hired for the sum of $20.00, for their "total extermination".[1]

Nor was the rate of pay likely to make amends for the living conditions. In speaking of the Contagious Disease Department, Dr. Kirkpatrick says: "It is extremely difficult to get respectable and trustworthy women to submit to the necessary isolation, even at $15.00 per month."

On October 12, 1889, Miss Rimmer resigned. Her health was not good, and in spite of efforts to retain her she would not continue. She died in 1892, of cancer, and the Committee of Management record a note of sincere gratitude for her services, as well as recognizing her striking personality.[2]

II

Immediately after Miss Rimmer's resignation the Medical Board urged upon the Committee of Management:

"That it is desirable that a certificated, trained nurse be appointed in the place of Miss Rimmer, and that such a person shall be selected with a view to her fitness to establish a training school for nurses."

It was quite evident now that the day of the untrained type of matron was past, and the demand for a training school was becoming insistent. The position was advertised both in the local papers and in American medical journals, stating that

"The candidate must be a certificated trained nurse, with experience of nursing in a general hospital, and must be fully competent to undertake at an early date the direction of a training school for nurses."

---

[1] Dr. F. G. Finley recalls seeing a rat drop off one of the pipes in the ceiling on to a patient's bed. Dr. F. S. Patch has described for me the rat hunts which used to be carried out in the basement rooms, with the help of dogs.

[2] Neither Miss Machin's nor Miss Rimmer's salaries are shown in the books. They both received remuneration, but by mutual agreement with the Committee the amount was not stated.

The first candidate was Miss E. A. Draper, of Chicago, who was unanimously recommended for the position by a committee of medical men. It is not certain whether she applied herself or not, as the Committee received a letter from her saying that she was "entirely in the dark as to the position offered me". She thought it would be better if she came to Montreal to investigate. This she did, and was received and entertained by Mr. F. W. Thomas and shown over the hospital. But within a few days she returned to Chicago and wired her refusal.[1]

Then the application of Miss Gertrude Elizabeth (Nora)[2] Livingston was considered. Miss Livingston was a graduate of the New York Hospital's Training School for Nurses. She had at first begun to train at the Mount Sinai Hospital, after having made an application to the New York Hospital which was not accepted because she did not present herself for a personal interview. She must, however, have given early proof of her unusual abilities as she attracted the attention during her probationary period of Mr. Ludlam and Miss Sutcliff, chairman and superintendent, respectively, of the New York Hospital. Mr. Ludlam through mutual friends finally arranged for her to come to his hospital, and after ten weeks at the Mount Sinai she began her training at the New York Hospital, whence she graduated in two years' time.

Miss Livingston was born in Sault Ste. Marie, Mich., on May 17, 1848, of English parentage. Her father had been a captain in the British army, but had gone into business after retiring from the service. He brought his family to live in Como, Que., where they had the Shepherd family as neighbours. Here it was that the lifelong friendship between Miss Livingston and Dr. F. J. Shepherd, began. It was Dr. Shepherd who persuaded her to apply for the superintendency. As will be seen from her letters (see Appendix A) Miss Livingston knew Montreal society well.

The Committee of Management at first was equally divided for and against accepting her application, and it was eventually left to the sub-committee, who wrote Miss Livingston as follows:

[1] Miss Draper eventually became the first Lady Superintendent of the Royal Victoria Hospital.

[2] "Nora" was not her baptismal name. It was evidently bestowed on her as a pet name by her family and she used it regularly; she was always referred to familiarly in the hospital (but not in her presence) by that name.

"I have the pleasure of informing you that your application for the position of lady superintendent of the M.G.H. has had the consideration of the committee, and their unanimous approval, and that I am authorized to offer you this position at a salary of $800.00 per annum . . . I believe you know the hospital and the duties of the position, but any information you require will be gladly given." January 21, 1890.

Miss Livingston wanted to know a great deal more. She replied as follows (January 24, 1890):

"I received your note this morning informing me of the favourable consideration and approval of my application. You offer no information regarding the duties of the position. Will you kindly let me know what is expected of me? Have I anything to do with the housekeeping? If I accept the position I ought to have at least two trained nurses chosen by myself, to act under me.

If you will allow me this, please inform me of the remuneration you would offer, so that I can make arrangements before leaving here. I could not possibly be in Montreal before the first week in February, as I am in charge of a critical case, and I could not leave before filling my place satisfactorily."

The president of the hospital, Mr. J. Stirling, replied to Miss Livingston, and, after expressing satisfaction at her taking the position, went on to say:

"The duties of the position are the engaging and discharging of all nurses and of all the female servants: the charge of the napery and the general superintendence of all that goes on in the Hospital, subject of course to the Committee of Management, whose unswerving support in everything they consider reasonable you may confidently depend upon. As for housekeeping, the Lady Superintendent will not have any of the work of that department to attend to. There always has been and will be a housekeeper to attend to all the details of that particular work.

The committee will allow you at least two trained nurses to act under you, but coming from the States do not know what remuneration they would expect. Our head nurses get $12.00 per month. Before committing themselves, the Committee would like to know about the customary rate of pay for trained nurses in the States, as I suppose they would expect as much here, and the probability seems to be that they will have to be got from the States . . ."

Miss Livingston replied:

"I have just received your note, which was quite satisfactory, with the exception of that part relating to the engaging and discharging of servants, as coming under the head of my duties. Now, in all successfully conducted hospitals, this comes strictly within the province of the housekeeper, and is considered the most trying and important duty of her position. Could not an arrangement be made that the housekeeper of the Montreal General Hospital undertake this, and so give me more time to bestow upon the all-important work of directing and teaching the nurses?

As to the remuneration expected by the trained nurses: I have talked the matter over with several superintendents and no properly certified nurse from an accredited school would go to Montreal under $30.00 per month. The price here is from that to $40.00, and would be difficult to obtain at that, as institutional work is only preferred by the few . ."

The president was then authorized to write Miss Livingston to engage two nurses and come without delay. He also told her that the handling of the servants would be left to the housekeeper. The number of beds in the hospital at the time was 165 and the nurses 30–35.

With regard to engaging the trained nurses, Miss Livingston **was** authorized to obtain two at a salary of about $30.00 per month **each**, but a few dollars more would be paid if necessary. Her final acceptance was as follows:

After agreeing to a salary of $800.00 per annum, with the hope of an increase "after we shall have mutually proved each other" she went on: "I shall leave here (D.V.) the middle of next week but I will telegraph you the exact day on which to expect me. I fear there will be great difficulty in getting suitable nurses; out of 11 nurses' names given me by the superintendent of the New York I have not yet secured one. The climate is a serious objection, and the distance from home and friends. The first of March would be as soon as we could expect to have them in Montreal, if we can get them at all."

Later Miss Livingston wrote that she would have to offer $35.00 each for two good nurses, and this was agreed to, but Mr. Stirling added:

"according to our ideas this appears to be big wages for nurses, and so I hope you will succeed in engaging them for somewhat less."

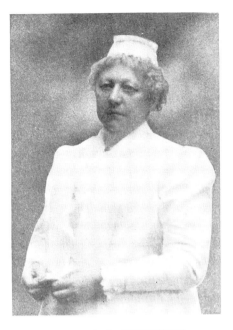

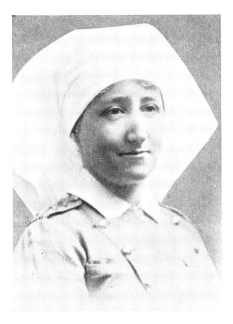

MISS N. G. E. LIVINGSTON   MISS S. E. YOUNG

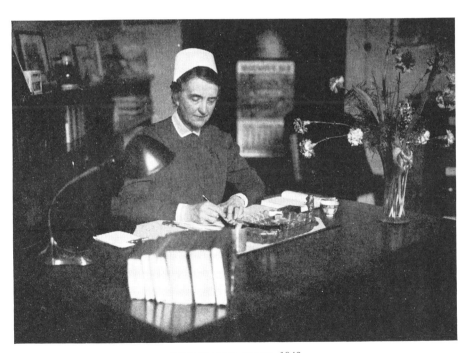

MISS MABEL HOLT, 1940

(Courtesy of *The Canadian Nurse*)

CHAPTER VI

The conditions which confronted Miss Livingston have been referred to by Dr. Shepherd as "Augean" and she herself in after years described them in no less forcible terms. Indeed, it is recorded that when she first visited the hospital on Dr. Shepherd's invitation, with a view to applying for its superintendency, her decision was an emphatic "Never", and only after considerable effort was she persuaded to apply for it.

Her account of conditions as given in later years is well described by Miss Frances Upton from details given her by Miss Livingston herself.

"On her arrival Miss Livingston found the front hall of the hospital papered with copies of the *London Illustrated News*; hospital linen drying everywhere. The heating system consisted of a large stove, which had but one leg, the three missing being supplemented by firebricks. In the children's ward, a curtain drawn across a portion of the wall covered up what turned out to be a case of diphtheria. There were no reports regarding patients' conditions, no medical lists, no medicine cupboards. Each patient helped himself from the bottle which reposed upon a shelf behind his bed—this shelf also contained his tobacco and his soap. Convalescents regularly helped prepare food in the kitchen.

There were no bed springs. Patients rested on straw mattresses or blankets, which were laid on a framework of iron pipes. Some were propped up on chairs. Typhoid fever patients were forced to get out of bed and drink the milk left in saucers in the middle of the floor, for cats. Dead bodies were wrapped in newspapers. Shrouds and mortuary baskets were unheard of. Miss Livingston asked the Committee for shrouds and they said to her, "How will we get them back?" But a special committee meeting was held and she won her point. In the outpatient department the gynæcological patients were attended by ward maids—it was much beneath the dignity of a nurse of that time to care for such patients. Miss Livingston had to insist on their doing this work.

Some of the immediate reforms brought about were: One hundred bed quilts and mattresses were ordered, and instructions were given to change the quilts when dirty. Chart boards were made to hang over the patients' beds, and this idea met with much opposition at first. Medicine lists were instituted and nurses were taught to compute and record doses, and to write reports and remarks, especially night orders. This, too, met with opposition at first. A fire system was established."

Miss Livingston arrived at the hospital on February 20, 1890.[1] Her two assistants, Miss Fanny Quaife and Miss Collyer, came on about two weeks later, and the training school started its work on April 1, 1890.

Then began the reign of one who not only laid the foundation but raised much of the superstructure of the present School. Miss Livingston was a born administrator. As was said of her by Earl Grey when visiting the hospital as Governor General, "she is a regular general". She had had no special training other than in general nursing, and her supervisory experience had been limited to being in charge of a large ward for the last two months of her course at the New York Hospital. But she knew exactly what she wanted, and what was equally important, knew the right things to want. She made no unreasonable demands, either on the hospital management or on the nurses, but she always was a firm disciplinarian. She began to ask for things very soon after she arrived, requesting, for example, that messengers should be provided to take medicines to the wards, instead of having her nurses waste their time on that kind of work. Some of her other requests to the Committee have already been mentioned.

A few of her rules for the School may be quoted:

HOUSE RULES

"(1) The hour for rising is 6 a.m. Before 11 a.m. each nurse must make her bed, dust and arrange her room, leaving it in good order, so that it may be ready for inspection at any hour thereafter.

(2) At 10 p.m. the light will be extinguished in the sitting room and corridors. The lights in the nurses' rooms must be out by 10.30 p.m. The gas must be turned down when the nurse leaves her room, even for the shortest time.

---

[1] This date is in accordance with the report made to the Committee by Dr. Kirkpatrick, the Superintendent. Miss Livingston says in her letters that it was the 22nd. She probably began work on that day.

(3) No visitors are to be invited to meals, or to spend the night on the premises. The sitting room may be used for the reception of visitors. A nurse may invite none but ladies to her room.

(8) On the entrance of an officer or stranger into the wards, nurses shall at once rise. All visitors must be given prompt attention."

The form of application for the school was as follows:

Candidate's name in full and address......................
Are you a single woman or a widow?.....................
      Note: Do not say 'Living at home'
Place and date of birth...............................
Height and weight....................................
Where educated......................................
Are you strong and healthy and have you always been so?....
Are your eyesight and hearing perfect?...................
Do you ever wear glasses? If so, for what reason?..........
Have you any tendency to pulmonary complaints?..........
Have you any physical defects?.........................
If a widow, have you any children? How many? How old?....
How are they provided for?............................
Where (if any) was your last situation? How long were you in it?..
Names in full and addresses of two persons to be referred to....
Have you ever been in any training school? If so, where?.....
Have you read and do you understand the regulations?....

Some idea of her maintenance of discipline may be gained from the following incidents. On one occasion the medical superintendent, Dr. Kirkpatrick, recommended to the Committee of Management that the nurses should be given white bread instead of brown. At the next Board meeting Miss Livingston supported the request. But she added that she had been unable to discover the nurses who complained about the bread, "but had cautioned them against carrying their grievances to outsiders, as such revelations were disloyal to the hospital and to the superintendents."

The Committee, it may be added, were divided in opinion about white bread for the nurses, but finally recommended that white sugar be supplied to the nurses' table.

On another occasion Miss Livingston reported to the Committee that:

"From lack of vigilance on the part of a nurse (Miss C. MacKay) a patient had escaped from the hospital, and

41

suggested that the nurse should be given the option of resigning or of serving a longer time."

The patient had escaped while Miss MacKay was at dinner, and it seems a little hard that the negligence should have been visited on her. However, it was resolved that she should have "the privilege of remaining in the school by a transfer to the senior class, involving a stay of three or four months longer." Miss MacKay was one of those who had taken most of their training under Miss Rimmer.

But Miss Livingston was continually thoughtful about the comfort of her nurses. The late Miss Julia English, one of the first graduates of the School, records that on one occasion when she and another nurse went to early service, her friend fainted in church, but went back on duty in the hospital. Miss Livingston heard of it and thereupon arranged to have tea and toast made for the nurses to have before they went to early service.

II

Cooking was not part of the training at first. In 1891 a school for cookery in the city offered to give lessons in the hospital, but the Committee would not agree to it. They felt that this work should be done by the nurses as part of their duty. Later on, another offer was made, the lessons to cost the hospital $20.00 for ten nurses, and the dishes made by the pupils to be bought by the hospital at cost. This plan was followed for a time. Later yet, Mr. F. Wolferstan Thomas had a dietitian brought out from England to give lessons to the nurses. She demonstrated, while they sat by. But this did not satisfy Miss Livingston, who had complaints about the food. At first she asked for a diet kitchen for private patients, but the Committee would not agree to that. Then she talked the matter over with Dr. Craik and finally persuaded the authorities to make the trial. There was one nurse in charge of this.

In 1897 Miss Livingston's sister, Miss Gracie, was appointed in charge of the diet kitchen, giving two hours a day instruction. This was later extended until the nurses came to spend two months of their time in the diet kitchen under Miss Gracie.

Until the new wing was added the diet kitchen occupied the space underneath one of the surgical wards (M). It was then moved to its present quarters on the 7th floor.

After Miss Gracie's retirement the teaching of dietetics was taken over by a trained dietitian, Miss Maude Perry. In addition to teaching the nursing staff a department of dietetics was gradually built up which gave a regular course in the subject for professional dietitians. This school is in charge of Miss Parkes. It operates independently of the nursing school, being directly responsible to the medical superintendent of the Hospital. Miss Gracie remained in charge until her retirement in 1919. The two sisters occupied the matron's suite.

The popularity of the School grew rapidly. In the first year Miss Livingston reported that there had been 160 applications. Eighty of these were entered on approbation; 42 of them proved satisfactory, four resigned for satisfactory reasons, and two were dismissed.

As regards uniforms, it was some time before the present pattern was decided on. Before Miss Livingston's arrival there had been a uniform for the nurses but they wore pretty much what they liked while on duty. As a rule their dress was of blue print, with a cap of book muslin made by themselves. After serving a year in the hospital they were allowed to put a black velvet ribbon on their caps.

Miss Livingston soon decided on a uniform, but the material itself was changed more than once. At first it was a pink and white striped pattern,[1] which was changed when the Royal Victoria Hospital also chose pink and white. Then a pink patterned material was chosen. This, however, was hurriedly changed again when Miss Livingston happened one day to notice that one of the orderlies was wearing a shirt of the same pattern, which he had acquired in a shop on the "Main Street"![2] Miss Livingston and Dr. Kirkpatrick then designed the present pattern with the Montreal General Hospital monogram.

---

[1] The Governors, in approving of this uniform, spoke of it as "a composition of pink and white gown with a neat cap and badge, all esthetic and antiseptic".

[2] Samples of these materials are preserved in the museum in the Nurses' Home.

At first the probationers had no special uniform, and then Miss Livingston introduced the plain blue dress and apron: the cap was granted at the end of three months.

An outdoor uniform was designed, with a dark cape and blue bonnet, with an Alsatian bow. Miss Livingston appeared before the Committee of Management in it. She said it would have a protective value for the nurses, and that the cost would be only $6.30. The Committee left it over for a while, and then decided that the hospital must not be involved in the cost. The nurses then bought the uniform themselves.

The first night nurse in charge engaged by Miss Livingston was a Miss Collyer of the New York Hospital School who was having a holiday before nursing. She came and tried it for a short time only. Then there was a nurse from the Edinburgh Infirmary who had come out here in straitened circumstances. Then came Mrs. Greatorex, an English graduate, who stayed about 18 months. She was personally attractive but lacked firmness. She was succeeded by Miss Baikie, one of the first graduates of the hospital, who stayed until Miss Jennie Webster began her long reign.

III

At this time Miss Livingston asked for and was granted a rise in salary to $1,000, but at the same time the Committee impressed on her "the necessity for economy".

Her first report on the school to the Committee made on August 11, 1890, was as follows:

> "There are 30 nurses, 17 of whom after serving two months' probation (without remuneration) have signed to remain for two years, subject to the rules and regulations of the training school. Six of the old nurses have joined the class, and with a year's training will receive their diplomas, their former services being accepted as equivalent to one year's work.
> "The next class to be organized this summer will be limited to twelve members; already there are 15 applicants for admission. The character of these candidates, their antecedents and education, render them worthy of confidence. Their capacity to become 'trained nurses' will be proved by their probationary term."

A letter from Miss Livingston to the president was also read, referring to the authority given her some weeks before to secure the services of two trained nurses, one to act as night nurse, and the other as day nurse, to replace the nurse who was then leaving. Miss Livingston had found it difficult to procure these nurses; one with good testimonials had proved unsuitable. There had been numerous applicants, but those of good standing objected to the lack of modern conveniences in the hospital and to defraying their travelling expenses.

In view of these difficulties Miss Livingston suggested that Miss Quaife, who was a thoroughly reliable "proved" nurse and could undertake the charge of the day work, should be engaged from September 1st, at a salary of $50.00 per month, as day nurse in charge. This was agreed to, but the Committee wanted it understood that it was an exceptional case, and was not to be considered as a precedent for the remuneration in future of anyone else engaged in the like capacity.

The members of this first graduating class were as follows: they are rightly referred to by Dr. Maude E. Abbott as "historic, for their graduation represents the establishment of a brilliant and fundamental reform".([1])

> Ellen Chapman
> Georgina Carroll
> Jessie M. Preston
> Julia English
> Christina Mackay
> Alicia Dunne

Miss Livingston in after years said that at first she was rather anxious about the prospects of this first graduating class. She had been laughed at for supposing that they would ever get the fee of $2.00 per day, which is what they were supposed to charge. Some people even asked her if the nurse could not also be made to do sewing for the family "when not attending to the patient"! The organization of the School was only part of Miss Livingston's task. She had to educate the public to recognize the higher standards she was setting up in nursing.

Until 1895 the course consisted of two years. In the spring of that year the first three-year course was initiated.

([1]) Lectures on The History of Nursing: p. 43.

The original curriculum of lectures was as follows:

Two lectures will be given on anatomy; prominence being given to the bones, arteries, nerves and surface markings.

Two lectures on materia medica including poisons and their antidotes.

Two on physiology.

One on dressings, instruments and appliances.

One on hygiene, ventilation, dietetics and disinfectants.

One on bandaging.

One on slight ailments and their treatments.

Two on medical emergencies such as, fits, unconsciousness, dyspnoea, internal hæmorrhage, and the use of the hypodermic syringe.

Two on Surgical Emergencies, embracing hæmorrhage, burns and scalds, accidents and their treatments.

One lecture on diseases of the eye and ear.

One on the throat and nose.

One on gynæcological nursing.

One on children's emergencies.

One on contagious diseases.

One on fever nursing and temperature taking.

Two on obstetrical nursing. In all twenty-two lectures.

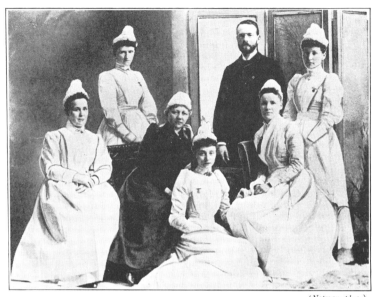

(*Notman photo*)

THE FIRST GRADUATES, WITH DR. R. C. KIRKPATRICK,
MEDICAL SUPERINTENDENT.

Standing (*left to right*): Miss Christina Mackay; Miss Georgina Carroll.
Seated: Miss Julia English, Miss Livingston, Miss Jessie Preston, Miss Quaife.

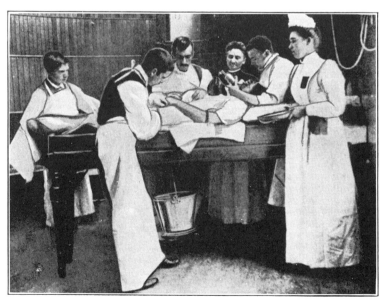

IN THE OLD OPERATING ROOM.

Dr. C. F. Martin is holding up the arm with the tourniquet on it. Opposite
is Dr. Harvey Smith, with Nurse Alicia Dunne looking on; she wore no
cap. The anæsthetist is Dr. Tait McKenzie.

CHAPTER VII

The graduation of the first class was a notable occasion. It was held on December 11, 1890, in the Windsor Hall (given without charge), and the Governor-General, Lord Stanley, came down from Ottawa to preside. The proceedings were prolonged, and by the time it was over the nurses must have been impressed, if not slightly dazed. Some extracts from the report of the proceedings may be of interest:

"Mr. John Stirling, president of the hospital, occupied the chair. On his left sat the Governor-General; on his right were Lady Stanley, Miss Clifton and Miss Livingston. On the platform were many leading citizens, including Sir William and Lady Dawson, Lady Smith, His Lordship Bishop Bond, Rev. Canon Ellegoode, Rev. H. J. Evans, Messrs. J. P. Cleghorn, R. W. Shepherd, Chas. Alexander, S. H. Ewing, J. C. Holden, John Crawford, Richard White, Chas. Garth, S. Finley, G. W. Stephens, F. Wolferstan Thomas, Sheriff Thibadeau, President, Notre Dame Hospital, Walter Drake, Professor Bovey, Dr. Craik, Dr. Hingston, Dr. McCallum and many others.
So soon as the audience was settled down a rustle was heard at the back of the hall, and the nurses attached at the training school entered in two columns, headed by Miss Quaife, the Assistant Superintendent, and Dr. Kirkpatrick, Medical Superintendent. Dressed in pretty pink dresses with long aprons and neat mob caps, white as the driven snow, they presented a most attractive appearance, and when they had taken their seats on raised platforms on each side of the hall, made up a picture worthy of an artist's brush. Their fresh complexions, neat attire, and evident enthusiasm for their work at once captivated the audience. It was interesting to notice how each nurse, despite the uniformity of their dress, had some individuality about her which distinguished her from her fellows. It may have been only a kink of the hair or some peculiar arrangement of the dress, yet each was distinguishable from the other by some mark of individual taste."

The meeting was opened by the Bishop of Montreal, after which Mr. Stirling gave a short account of the growth of the hospital. The nurses after this settled down to listen to a long address by Dr. McCallum. Lord Stanley then spoke. At one point he reminded the nurses "They should be careful, while effecting the cure of a patient, that they did not leave incipient cases of heart disease behind". Dr. Craik followed, as representing the Committee of Management, and the proceedings closed with the benediction.

The complete roll of the training school at this time was as follows:

Head Nurses

Miss Ellen Chapman
Miss Georgina Carroll
Miss Jessie M. Preston
Miss Julia English
Miss Christina MacKay

Senior Assistants

Miss Eliz. Baikie
Miss Alma E. Bush
Miss Barbara Haggart
Miss Bessie Conner
Miss Charlotte M.
  Hetherington
Miss Ethel Hobday
Miss Annie Colquhoun
Miss Maggie Jackson
Miss Alice Cashen
Miss Eleanor Sait
Miss Annie S. Prime
Miss Hattie Howes
Miss Emily Cooper
Miss Ellen Thompson
Miss Edith M. Green
Mrs. Marie O'Donovan

Junior Assistants

Miss Eugenie Burton
Miss Mary Collins
Miss Adelaide F. Seaton
Miss Emma C. Mercer
Miss Effie Darling
Miss Angie Dancey
Miss Alice M. Hall
Miss Jessie McGregor
Miss Jean Sinclair
Miss Sallie Foster
Miss Nora Jolly
Miss Mary Annand

Day Nurse in Charge

Miss Fannie Quaife

Night Nurse in Charge

Mrs. Greatorex

Nurse in Charge of O.R.

Miss Alicia Dunne

In the following year the graduation ceremonies were held with rather less formality in the Natural History Hall. The newspaper account allowed itself some facetious comments:

"Away down at the back of the hall a group of medical students testified their interest in the proceedings by frequent outbursts of applause. In the front row sat the graduating class of the training school, 11 in number. On each side were the undergraduates. All were arrayed in the pretty pink costume and white coat of the school. It might be incidentally remarked that the costumes were not the only things that were pretty! There was a McGill flavour about the proceedings, which opened with prayer."

Miss Livingston had to strive for additional nurses, the Committee being always difficult to convince on this point. It was felt that there should be a special nurse in charge of the operating room used by Drs. Gardner, Alloway and Buller, representing gynæcology and ophthalmic work, and she proposed paying her $25.00 per month. At first the Committee demurred. They proposed that one of the ordinary nurses should do the work, at $12.00 per month.

However, later on, it was agreed to have a nurse to look after this special operating room at $25.00 monthly, but she must be one of the training school, and would also do the work of an ordinary nurse there.

The ordinary operating room was in charge of Miss Alicia Dunne, who had been there before Miss Livingston's arrival. She was a woman of unusual personality, and Miss Livingston had been carefully warned before she took charge "Whatever you do, don't quarrel with Alicia".[1] It does not appear that there was ever any friction. Nurse Alicia resigned in 1897,[2] and was succeeded by Miss Nora Tedford.

I am indebted to Miss Nora Tedford for the following reminiscences of Miss Dunne.

"Miss Dunne had been trained under Dr. Roddick and Dr. Fenwick. She was a fine looking woman, tall, silvery-haired, witty. Her bed-sitting room, which was behind what is now the main operating room and is now being used for the nose and throat work, was frequently visited by young internes, who liked to get her point of view; perhaps also a little supper.

---

[1] Before Miss Livingston's advent, nurses were usually addressed by their Christian names, e.g., "Nurse Alicia". Miss Livingston, however, preferred the use of surnames, and this became customary.

[2] Nurse Alicia was one of those who was given a medal and certificate after one year in the School. Miss Livingston's comment on her, in her private record of nurses, was: "Clear, capable, dignified. *Difficult* temper."

Nurse Alicia always dined alone, her meals being sent in to her from the main kitchen. She wore no cap, and always had on a stiffly starched gingham uniform, spotless and with elbow length white cuffs. She gave a good training according to the times. Always washed and sterilized her hands, but wore no gloves or sterilized costume. She had survived the days when the operating room was drenched with antiseptic irrigations, and the use of the antiseptic steam kettle. She saw the change from all this to the dry technique fostered largely by Dr. Shepherd."

Dr. A. T. Bazin has also contributed some notes from his personal memories of Miss Dunne.

His first contact with her was as a second year student when in the best tradition of the day he became sick and faint whilst watching his first operation. Dr. Shepherd, the surgeon, merely told him to stretch out on the bench, whilst Nurse Alicia gave him a smile of encouragement.

"Her expression was kindly, but when roused her eyes would flash and her chin would set. She never raised her voice, but her words and tone would cut scathingly. The needless infliction of pain would at once rouse her ire.

Her two heroes on the staff were Dr. Roddick, because of the tender gentleness of his touch, and Dr. Shepherd, because of his honest dealings.

When Miss Livingston became Superintendent in 1890, Nurse Alicia was firmly in the saddle as nurse in charge of the operating room, and the formalities of Miss Livingston's visits to the operating room suite were parallel to those of the King of England when proceeding to or through the City of London.

Miss Livingston would approach the door to Nurse Alicia's 'office' and there stand until the latter would appear, when the formal inspection would proceed. If Nurse Alicia were not available at the time, the inspection would be postponed.

She would never ally herself with the training school, not because she was opposed to it, but because she considered she belonged to other times and customs.

I was and am proud of being classed by her as 'one of my b'yes'. She was born and educated in Quebec and had a delightful brogue.

For many years she lived in this city with her niece— Miss O'Reilly—a graduate nurse of a New York Hospital. On the death of the latter she broke up the household and went back to her native city of Quebec, where she lived with a former schoolmate, Mrs. Rooney. I repeatedly visited her both in Montreal and Quebec. She finally died at a ripe old age, the actual count of years remaining a secret, alike to the records of the hospital and her friends."

II

One of the most pressing developments in the growth of the training school was the need for a nurses' home. Miss Livingston interested herself in it very keenly, and urged continually that a home should be built. The matter had been under discussion for a long time, but now the need had become acute. Complaints were made more than once that the sleeping quarters of the nurses were infested with bugs and rats, and Mr. Mould, the steward, reported to the Committee that he found three rooms with insects in them. Besides, the nurses were increasing in number, and more space was needed. A mansard roof had been added to the main building soon after Miss Livingston's arrival, and this had served as nurses' quarters. But it had become inadequate.

But even Miss Livingston's energy and determination would have failed to bring about this object without the help of others. Fortunately, Mr. Wolferstan Thomas, one of the hospital's most notable benefactors, interested himself in the plan. He wrote to the newspapers about it and aroused public support. On one occasion he gave a dinner to a large number of his friends. When Mr. Thomas rose to speak, someone said to his neighbour, "Frank is on his begging legs again". But the dinner had been so unusually good that the ground was well prepared and "Frank's" appeal for funds was well responded to. At last, in 1896 the necessary funds were raised and the building was begun. It was called the Jubilee Nurses' Home, in commemoration of Queen Victoria's Diamond Jubilee, and on September 2, 1897, the foundation stone was laid by Lord Lister, who happened to be in Canada for a meeting of the British Association. He has left his signature in the Governors' Visiting Book. It was fitting that the chairman of the proceedings should be Dr. Thomas Roddick, who had been not only one of the foremost surgeons on the staff of the hospital (he was at the time the chief surgeon at the Royal Victoria Hospital), but also the first to introduce Lord Lister's methods of antisepsis into the Montreal General Hospital.[1]

This building has now been overshadowed by a nurses' residence (even the word "home" has been supplanted!), built 30 years later on the ground facing the hospital on Dorchester Street. Although Miss Livingston had retired long before this further expansion, she lived to see the new building opened. But we may doubt whether it could have given her any greater pleasure and sense of accomplishment than did the original home. She saw her nurses properly housed, in a new building with ample space, and an atmosphere of refinement and comfort which contributed much to the success of the school.[2]

---

[1] The antiseptic spray originally brought from England by Dr. Roddick has been presented to the hospital by Dr. W. Turner, to whom it had been given by Dr. Roddick.

[2] It may be noted here that Miss Livingston was responsible for obtaining in 1911 a donation from Mr. Sherringham Shepherd of $5,000 for defraying expenses of nurses in training needing special vacations after illness. This amount was supplemented by a further £1,000 under the terms of Mr. Shepherd's will in 1920.

CHAPTER VIII

For the first 15 years the school carried on a very thorough course of training, following fairly closely on the lines laid down first by Miss Livingston. This included theoretical and practical training, with most emphasis on the latter. The programme submitted to the Board of Management by Miss Livingston in 1900 was as follows:

LENGTH OF COURSE—3 Years

Division of time for practical experience in the various branches of nursing.
Surgical ....10 months⎫ Six months of which is night duty
Medical..................10 months⎭
Out Department.......... 3 months
Operating Theatres........ 3 months
Gynæcology.............. 4 months
Private patients........... 1 month
Diet kitchen.............. 2 months
Vacation................. 9 weeks—being 3 weeks each year.
Length of scholastic year—from October 1st to June 1st.

CLASSES

Divided into four classes, as follows:
>Head Nurses
>Senior Nurses
>Junior Nurses
>Probationers

Textbooks used:
>Weeks' Manual—General Nursing.
>Kimber's Anatomy and Physiology.

Notes on special diseases and emergencies—Miss Livingston.

Instructors:
Head Nurses................Miss Livingston..........Tuesday, 7.15 p.m.
Head Nurses................Miss Livingston..........Thursday, 7.15 p.m.
Seniors....................Miss Livingston..........Thursday, 2.30 p.m.
Seniors....................Miss McLean............
Juniors....................Miss Shaw..............Friday, 7.15 p.m.
Bandage class..............Miss Baikie.............Wednesday, 7.15 p.m.
Practical pharmacy..........Mr. W. P. Watson........Monday, 7.15 p.m.
Lecture by member of Medical
   Board ....Saturday, 8.00 p.m.
Diet Kitchen, Practice and
   Theory................Miss G. Livingston.......Friday, 7.00 p.m.

Examinations:

Are held at the end of every year, conducted by a member of the Medical Board. This examination is both written and oral. 'Ward Marks' for practical work and deportment are included in the general average.

What merits a diploma?

General excellence in examinations, deportment and work.([1])

As time went on, however, Miss Livingston began to realize the great value of giving the nurses more preliminary training before they actually began their ward work. This, however, meant extra instruction and she was unable to put her idea into operation for some time. At last, in 1906, she gained her object. In her report for February 21 of that year she records that

> "through the liberal gift of a member of the Committee of Management,([2]) a new and important feature of training would be introduced next September, that of a preliminary course for probationers under a competent instructor, thus giving the probationer a knowledge of her work before she applies it."

The "competent instructor" in this work was Miss Flora Madeline Shaw,([3]) one of the notable figures associated with the development of the school. Miss Shaw was a native of Perth, Ont., where she was born in 1864, graduating from the M.G.H. in 1896. She must have shown early in her work her unusual capacities for teaching, for she became Miss Livingston's second assistant as soon as she graduated. After three years in this position she took charge of a small woman's hospital in Boston, returning to the hospital in 1900 as first assistant to Miss Livingston until 1903.

Miss Shaw continually widened her knowledge and experience. Between 1904 and 1906 she attended the Teacher's College of Columbia University and received her diploma for "Teaching in Schools of Nursing". In 1906 she again returned to Miss Livingston to take charge of the probationary class, as mentioned. She acted in this capacity until January 1909, when she was forced by illness

---

([1]) Miss Livingston's note in her "Nurses' Record Book" reads: "During the two years' course nurses received a vacation of four weeks. 'Lost time', either from illness or imperative claims must be made up."

([2]) Mr. Reid Wilson.

([3]) An excellent description of the methods followed in these preliminary classes is given by Miss Shaw in the Proceedings of the Second Annual Convention of Canadian Society of Superintendents of Training Schools for Nurses, Ottawa, 1908, p. 49.

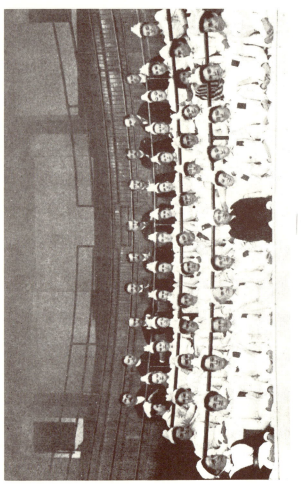

CLASS OF 1892.

Probably the only instance in which the house surgeons were photographed along with the nursing staff. Those in the back row are: Mr. Bates, the steward; Dr. W. W. Matson; Dr. C. F. Martin; Dr. Harvey Smith; Dr. W. F. Hamilton; Dr. Tait McKenzie; Dr. H. B. Carmichael; ————; Dr. Hewitson.

to retire from active work.([1]) This ended her direct connection with the hospital, but in 1920 she accepted the position as Directress of the School for Graduate Nurses at McGill University upon its foundation. This position she held until her death. The school was one of Miss Shaw's dearest interests.

Judged by mere passage of time Miss Shaw's service to the hospital was not very long. But she left an abiding mark in the school. She was really a pioneer in the branches of the nursing field in which she was engaged, and came to be recognized as one of the most distinguished leaders and authorities in connection with nursing education in Canada. She was also internationally known and respected in the nursing world. She died on August 27, 1927, in Liverpool, after a very brief illness on her return from the interim congress of the International Council of Nurses at Geneva.

II

A brief reference to changes in the hospital itself will now be necessary. The completion of the nurses' home in 1896 had been preceded by the addition of two large wings to the hospital, devoted mainly to surgical wards, but containing also a children's ward and a floor for private patients. A large operating room and quarters for the medical staff were also provided. There had also been much remodelling of the old central building to provide extra space for the medical services and specialties.

In time, however, the necessity became pressing for further enlarging the medical side and for taking care of the growing outdoor department, as well as to provide more private wards and operating rooms. A suggestion that the whole hospital be moved to a site further uptown, on Ontario Street, was brought forward, but the idea was given up and it was decided to build an addition to the existing building. This took the form of a large seven-story building,([2]) providing for a large expansion in medical beds and

---

([1]) Miss Shaw was succeeded by Miss F. Strumm, who acted until 1916, when she took Miss Young's place as first assistant. Miss Ketchen followed Miss Strumm, and served until 1920, when Miss Rayside and Miss M. Holt became instructresses.

([2]) The plans provided for another similar wing on the west side of the hospital.

outdoor service, with space for an X-ray department, and private wards. This was opened in 1913, and raised the total bed capacity of the hospital to 425.

All this development meant increased demands on the nurses, and a growing staff, but Miss Livingston still showed herself entirely capable of steady, wise administration. It is to be noted that she never travelled or attended any conventions or gatherings of nursing bodies. But she fully realized the value to be derived from them and would always send representatives from her staff to attend them. In spite of her advancing years she was as active as ever, and with her intuitive powers and ceaseless personal supervision there was very little that escaped her notice. At the same time she had gathered about her a staff who very thoroughly absorbed her ideals and methods, whilst maintaining their own independence of personality. Miss Livingston was forceful and imperious, sometimes to the point of being high-handed, but she never suppressed freedom of expression in others. In fact, she welcomed it.

Miss Sarah E. Young, her assistant, was one of these. It would be difficult to imagine a more striking contrast than was presented by these two. Miss Livingston, quick, confident, dominating (but not domineering): Miss Young, quiet, almost to the point of diffidence, but equally tenacious of purpose and clear of vision.

A third figure on the staff was different again—Miss Flora Strumm, who is still active in the service of the hospital as assistant superintendent. Miss Strumm has a unique record of service. She has been assistant to three successive superintendents, and has acted as a coordinating link between the old and the new, tiding over each change in administration, and making possible a continuity of work which has been invaluable. Her capacities have lain not only in administration but in complete devotion to duty, and an unruffled sweetness of temper which is recognized by everyone in the institution.

To these must be added the name of Miss Nora Tedford, who for twenty-one years (1898-1919) not only shared in the teaching through her thorough training of nurses in the operating room, but set an example of gentleness and self-effacement which was of immeasurable influence in the School.

The night superintendent's work was carried on by one who created a unique record of service in the hospital—Miss Jennie Webster. Graduating in 1895, Miss Webster first acted as matron (for two and a quarter years) to the infectious hospital, which had finally been separated in that year from the hospital and moved to Moreau St. A short period of private nursing followed, but Miss Webster had always kept closely in touch with her school, and when Miss Baikie left in 1900 Miss Livingston at once sent for "Webster".

In no instance was Miss Livingston's choice more completely justified. Miss Webster took to her nocturnal occupation with perfect readiness and adaptation. The work called for both initiative and a capacity for very hard work. Both of these Miss Webster had in a marked degree. From the medical point of view her physical endurance was all the more remarkable in view of the fact that she had had rheumatic fever as a child, with a second attack during her training.

Miss Webster also had the ability to get people of the most diverse nature to do what she wanted them to do. For many years she had not only to carry on actual nursing of the patients, but also to deal with emergencies and situations requiring tact, firmness and quick decision. If there ever was any delay in a house surgeon being called to an emergency at night it certainly was not Miss Webster's fault. She treated the medical staff with a mixture of motherliness and deference which was hard to resist (even if one should want to!), but no one was ever exempt from her urgent personal summons at night when occasion arose.

In no respect did her powers show to better advantage (indeed she probably enjoyed it more than any other part of her work) than in the Out-patient Department. The best description of her is in Dr. Keith Gordon's finely executed sketch of her life.[1] Unfortunately, I can only quote from it very briefly:

> "When the walking sick that crowd the out-patient clinics during the hours of daylight have departed, and only a dim light burns here and there throughout the wards, it might appear to the casual observer that the hospital had gone to sleep, but this impression is soon dispelled if a visit is paid to that region where Miss Webster has begun to

[1] *The Canadian Nurse:* 1933; *29;* 235.

receive her blood-soaked and belligerent guests; for at this hour the brothels and dark streets of an unsavoury neighbourhood have begun to cast up their wreckage.

The arrival at the hospital of this type of patient is invariably attended by a morbidly inquisitive mob and a great deal of shouting on the part of the injured warriors and their seconds. Efforts on the part of a group of hospital orderlies to quell the riot are unsuccessful and only on the appearance of a very efficient-looking woman does order reign. The crowd disappears as if by magic and the patient becomes at once docile and even amicable. . .

There are again those who come to call upon her under pretext of some physical infirmity, and with a faint hope in their hearts that she may be persuaded to offer them a comfortable bed for the night, but her diagnosis of the true condition is seldom wrong. Conspicuous among this type of visitor is a gentleman by the name of Jimmie Cochrane, who at regular intervals makes his presence known by throwing his cap on the floor and proceeding to utter a series of shrill cries until Miss Webster arrives and solemnly inspects an imaginary disease of the foot, feeling perhaps that she can never compensate him for the loss of an artificial eye which she once destroyed while attending to his needs in the Outdoor."

On May 14, 1925, Miss Webster celebrated her 25th anniversary as night superintendent. Amidst the many letters which she received on that occasion was one from Miss Livingston herself, now aged and partially crippled, but with mental vigour undimmed. It read as follows:

"My dear Miss Webster:

Many happy returns of the day. It seems but yesterday that we made final arrangements for your entering on your duties as night superintendent—a trust which you have never betrayed. What a record!

Goodbye. God bless you.

G. E. N. Livingston."

Miss Webster's long period of service came to an end in January, 1933, when she retired to private life to look after two nephews who had suddenly lost their parents. Her leaving was the occasion for many evidences of the high regard in which she was held. As Dr. Gordon describes it:

"Perhaps the greatest tribute to the high esteem in which she was held was a reception given by the members of the training school, and which throngs of citizens in all walks of life attended, even to a representative from the Montreal Police Force."

Miss Webster was succeeded by Miss Christina Denovan.

III.

During the Great War no change was made in the course of training, although in 1914 Miss Livingston was induced to make one concession to its exigencies which may be mentioned. The nurses of the class for that year still had a few weeks to complete at the time war was declared, but certain members of the class[1] were so anxious to get into action overseas that they applied for military service before their graduation. They were told that they must be graduates before their applications could be considered, and they therefore appealed to Miss Livingston to hold the examinations immediately, in order to allow them to qualify. It actually was not a matter of more than a couple of weeks, and Miss Livingston readily granted their request. Legend has it that the ink was barely dry on their examination papers before these four nurses appeared at military headquarters again, to assure the authorities that they were now eligible. They left with the first contingent for England.

Otherwise, the work of the school was carried on as usual. Miss Young went overseas on military service in 1916, and Miss Strumm acted as first assistant. There was great difficulty in obtaining personnel for the work of the hospital during the war. House surgeons were few, and competent orderlies often could not be obtained. And yet the number of patients showed no diminution. The culmination of the strain came in 1918 when the epidemic form of influenza broke out in Montreal. During this period the medical and nursing professions generally were taxed to the uttermost, and the hospital was overcrowded with cases.

---

[1] Isabella Strathy, Juliette Pelletier, Georgina Massy and Marjorie Webb.

After the outbreak had subsided the Medical Board sent the following resolution to Miss Livingston:

> "The Medical Board of the Montreal General Hospital wishes to put on record their appreciation of the efficient manner in which the Lady Superintendent and her staff of graduate and undergraduate nurses have carried on the work of the hospital notwithstanding the enormous strain put upon the nursing staff by the unprecedented conditions of the present epidemic of influenza.
>
> In view of the great increase of work resulting from the overcrowding of the hospital and the reduction in the number of nurses from the large proportion who themselves contracted the disease, the devotion to duty displayed by the members of the training school under these conditions will always redound to the credit of the hospital.
>
> The Medical Board desires to extend its deepest sympathy to the relatives and friends of the nurses who succumbed in the discharge of their duty."

With the coming of peace, the work of the hospital immediately began to expand again. Miss Livingston carried on her work with no apparent alteration in energy, but in 1919 she developed a paralytic stroke. In spite of a fair recovery it was plain that she could not continue active work, and on her resignation the Board unhesitatingly appointed Miss Young in her place.

After her retirement, Miss Livingston lived quietly with her sister, Miss Gracie, until her death on July 24, 1927. Her mind remained active to the end, and she always maintained a keen interest in her "girls". The funeral service was held at Christ Church Cathedral, and she was buried in Como. A marble slab has been erected over her grave by the Alumnae Association.

IV

It is not easy to keep this account from becoming a life of Miss Livingston. In effect, the School *was* her life. It certainly was her creation, and she has left on it so strong an impress of her personality, that it would be a well merited tribute to devote its history mainly to her.

Naturally, however, consideration must be given to other personalities who have played and are playing valuable and important parts in the life of the School.

No special attempt has been made to gather reminiscences of Miss Livingston. Space will not permit of all that are at hand. Her nature and many of her characteristics will become apparent in the story of her work. The extracts from her letters given in Appendix A, perhaps, tell us more of her than any set description.

My own recollection of her, as a house surgeon in 1913, and as a student in the hospital before that, is of her unusual capacity for getting around to every corner of an irregularly laid out series of buildings, without haste and certainly with no apparent rest. She was stout in build, but there was nothing deliberate or portly in her manner, only a natural dignity which was never impaired. Her penetrating eyes missed nothing, but she was quite above prying. Possibly she realized, as she says in one of her letters, that in time everything becomes known in a hospital, but she was entirely straightforward in her methods. Furthermore, she had an exceedingly dry but acute sense of humour, and if she was apt, as Dr. Shepherd said of her, not "to suffer fools gladly", she extracted much fun from attempts to deceive her, which were numerous but seldom successful.

One of the nurses who trained under Miss Livingston and saw much of her in her years of retirement has kindly permitted me to include some of her own recollections.

"Miss Livingston always wore a gold chain at her waist with her keys on it. She would rattle these as she walked, intentionally. She hated to seem to be prying on people, and was willing to give them warning of her approach—'and they were fools if they did not take it' she would say.

She also wore at her waist a gold medal which had been given her by a very sick patient whom she had nursed in the Sloane Hospital in New York. 'Wear this always, and you will never catch any infectious disease', the patient told her (it was a religious medal and had been blessed by the Pope). Whatever its value, Miss Livingston always said that she escaped every infectious disease, although very much exposed at times. (In one of her letters she speaks of having no fear at all of any infection.)

Miss Livingston was never deceived by those who tried to hoodwink her, but she would never let on that she knew. One Sunday evening she found a nurse cooking something in the ward kitchen. 'What are you making, nurse?' 'Oh, I am just making some cocoa for a sick patient, Miss Livingston.' 'The fool' said Miss Livingston later on, 'as if I could not see it was fudge she was making for a couple of housemen whom I knew were waiting out on the gallery. What would she have said if I had asked her to let me taste it? And then when I went out and spoke to the housemen, one of them said, 'We're just waiting to see a sick patient'—as if all the patients weren't sick!'

Once, on the request of the superintendent of the day, she called in a nurse and gave her extra time as punishment for something she had done to offend the doctor. 'How I hated him for making me punish her,' she said.

While Nurse —— was in charge of the private wards, the report was made to Miss Livingston that she had far more linen on her ward than any other nurse in the hospital. Late one Sunday evening she heard the familiar rattle of the keys at the door of the ward, and there was Miss Livingston. 'Well, nurse, they tell me you have too much linen on your ward. How much have you?' 'Well, Miss Livingston, I have 130 sheets and so on, but I always keep my patients in fresh linen, and change them as often as I can.' 'You are quite right, nurse. You have a private ward, and must keep the linen fresh. But that is rather a lot to have. Suppose we take ten sheets from you, and let it go at that.' And then she told how, when she was a charge nurse herself in the Sloane Hospital, New York, she used to take the linen out of the ward cupboards and hide it in her own room, so as to have it to give to the patients, because she could not get enough for fresh changes for them otherwise."

Miss Livingston lost most of her family jewellery in 1915. It was stolen from her apartments one day when both she and Miss Gracie were out, and Sarah her maid was off for the day. The theft caused a stir at the time, and was referred to by Father Cotter, the visiting priest of the Jesuit order, as "The theft of the crown jewels". He always spoke of Miss Livingston as "Queen Victoria".

CHAPTER IX

Miss Young took over the superintendency with a very intimate knowledge and understanding of the work of the School. From the very beginning of her work she showed that whilst maintaining the high standards of the School she understood the trend towards less exacting working conditions.

First of all it was realized that the hours of work were too long, and the time off duty was therefore increased from one hour per day to three hours, in addition to the half day off per week already permitted.

Then came the lightening of much of the heavy ward work which, even if not excessive, was recognized as being a waste of time for nurses. In 1921 there appeared for the first time subsidiary workers on the wards (ward helpers), who did much of the routine mechanical work previously done by the nurses.

During the war the instructress work, which had been begun by Miss Shaw, had lapsed to some extent, and whilst the teaching and lecturing had been carried on, there was no special instructress. In 1920, however, new and improved methods of teaching were introduced. To begin with, the time-honoured system of doing all the teaching in the evenings was abandoned. Then, two new instructresses were engaged, who not only were able to carry on this work in the day, but also exercised more supervision of the nurses. These were Miss E. C. Rayside and Miss Mabel K. Holt.

It was in this year also that the formal graduation exercises were resumed. These had not been carried on for several years, the nurses being merely handed their medals as they graduated. These exercises are now an event in the calendar of the School.

In 1923, one of the most striking innovations in the history of the School was initiated. This was the inauguration of a system of student government, by which the internal discipline of the School was left largely to the students themselves. It was a change which could hardly have been expected in Miss Livingston's time. She had had to bear the responsibility of building up the School

63

herself, and when it reached its full development she was not prepared to change her methods. The change may be regarded as a
natural development of independence, or as the expression of a
sense of "self-determination" brought about by the ferment of the
war period. In any case, the demand for it was insistent, and Miss
Young had the wisdom to deal with it sympathetically.

On October 15, 1923, therefore, the Student Government
Association of the Montreal General Hospital came into being.
It was an organization consisting entirely of undergraduate nurses,
the officers being appointed solely by themselves. It was granted
power

> "to deal with all matters concerning the life and conduct of
> the student when off duty, to increase the feeling of co-
> operative unity amongst the students, and to establish a high
> standard of honour in all things pertaining to the life of the
> School."

The first president of this Association was Miss Grace Tanner,
and much of the credit for its formation is due to her. She held
office for only four months before graduating, and was succeeded
by Miss Gladys Buzzell, who had been treasurer. Miss Buzzell's
work was outstanding, and undoubtedly was a large factor in
carrying the Association through its difficult early years.

The benefits of the new method were not long in being realized,
both by the student body and by the administrative officers of the
hospital, from whom was lifted the burden of ceaseless watching
and admonition. The social life of the nurses and their recreational
opportunities were also greatly improved. The method is no longer
on trial. It is well established and works well.

Another change of note at this time was the introduction of
the system of having graduate nurses in charge of the wards,
instead of these being in the hands of a senior undergraduate.
This tended to lift some of the heavy responsibility which the
nurse in training was made to carry.

II

By this time, the problem of housing the nursing staff was
again becoming acute. In 25 years the Jubilee Nurses' Home had

become totally inadequate for the demands on its living and teaching quarters. How acute the need was may be judged by the fact that during Miss Young's term of office the teaching staff was trebled, and the various developments mentioned caused a sharp increase in the numbers of those living on the premises. In 1921 it was necessary to open a home for night nurses in a building at the corner of Ste. Famille and Sherbrooke St., but this was only a temporary measure.

A large new building was required, and this was finally obtained through a generosity and fineness of spirit on the part of the Board of Governors which is notable even amongst the many other splendid gifts to the hospital at various times. This generosity was well implemented by the Provincial Government, which gave a grant of $200,000 towards the cost of the building. The leading spirit in the whole enterprise was the late Colonel Herbert Molson, who was the president of the hospital at the time. His energy, generosity, and influence were unremittingly devoted to this extremely important development in the life of the School. It is not too much to say that without such a building the work of the School would have been impaired and retarded. With it, developments have been possible along modern lines, whilst always maintaining the high standards originally set by Miss Livingston.

The Home stands directly opposite the entrance to the hospital on Dorchester Street. It was formally opened in 1926 by the Honorable Taschereau, who was then Premier of the Province of Quebec.

In this building are housed all the permanent as well as the undergraduate members of the nursing staff. It contains a feature which it had always been Miss Young's ambition to achieve, that is, a complete teaching unit of laboratories and class rooms, all on one floor.

Miss Young only lived to see one year of its usefulness. She died on December 4, 1927.

It is in keeping with her nature that there is little to record of Miss Young herself, except the impression she left of a strong but retiring character. She was born in Quebec in 1877, and was educated in a private school before undertaking her training at the Montreal General Hospital in 1897. After graduating as head of her class she did private nursing for a short time, before returning to the hospital to become second assistant to Miss Livingston.

Miss Young was one of the few nurses on the active militia list when war broke out, but in spite of her desire to serve she was retained in the hospital until 1916, when she was released for military duty. She served a short time in England and then went to France where she was attached to No. 1 Canadian General Hospital, one of the largest and busiest hospitals in France. For her conspicuous and notable services she was awarded the Royal Red Cross.

In 1917 she was recalled to Canada to become matron of the Tuxedo Military Hospital in Winnipeg, and served as principal district matron of the area until her return to Montreal to take the place of Miss Livingston.

At the time of her death, Miss Young was only fifty years of age, but her influence in the development of the School was out of all proportion to the short length of her regime. Her modesty of manner, serenity of mind, and devotion to her work were only to be fully appreciated by those who were associated with her. She displayed always true religion and virtue, both in her work and daily life, and in her unfailing attendance at church.

III

Miss Young was succeeded by the present superintendent, Miss Mabel K. Holt. Miss Holt graduated from the School in 1919, in the last class under Miss Livingston's regime. After a short period of private nursing she joined the staff as first assistant to Miss Young, and in the following year became instructress. A further year of study was spent at the School for Graduate Nurses, McGill University, after which she returned to her own school as instructress in 1924. She then accepted an appointment as assistant superintendent of nurses at the Hamilton General Hospital. She was recalled to the hospital on account of Miss Young's illness in 1927, and in December of the same year was appointed as Lady Superintendent of the School.

The problems facing Miss Holt were rather different to those with which her predecessors had to deal. The School was now running on well organized lines, with an adequate building and no lack of applicants for the classes. But from 1930 onwards the critical years of the economic depression had a serious effect on the nursing profession in the city. So urgent did this problem become that there arose a danger of the lowering of hard-won educational standards.

However, in 1935, the Private Patients' Pavilion was added to the Western Division of the hospital, and in its opening Miss Holt saw an opportunity not only for providing the best possible nursing facilities, but also for relieving what had become an urgent problem of unemployment amongst graduate nurses. On Miss Holt's initiative the Committee of Management was persuaded to permit the staffing of the new wing entirely with graduate nurses, on the eight-hour plan. By this means, patients who were unable to afford individual private nurses were assured of attention which was practically continuous, and a large number of graduates found regular employment. The plan has worked smoothly from the beginning.

In 1937, a public health nurse was appointed with special responsibility for the development of a complete health service for student nurses, as well as for the integration of preventive aspects through the undergraduate course.

The expansion of the School may be regarded as complete so far as numbers are concerned, but the course of teaching keeps pace with the changing demands of the day. There is a great contrast, of course, between the training of the nurses in Miss Livingston's early years and that given the nurse of today, but any comparisons of this sort are not to be made with the idea of showing superiority so much as normal development. The 21 lectures provided in the early days have been replaced by a curriculum in keeping with modern requirements. The staff of three graduates and 38 student nurses of 1890 has grown into an organization headed by a Lady Superintendent who is also Principal of the School, a day and a night assistant; four full time instructresses; 45 graduate nurses; and 210 students. More than 1,600 nurses have been granted the diploma of the School.

The School has a dual function. It carries on a course of

training in general nursing, and it also provides a nursing staff for the care of the patients in the hospital.

Whilst the training in general nursing is as complete as may be desired, it has always been recognized that it had to be supplemented by education in aspects of medicine not included in the work of the hospital. As regards maternity work, the nurses at first spent two months at the Maternity Hospital, which later was increased to three. Curiously enough, maternity work as such is not mentioned in Miss Livingston's earlier curriculum.

The teaching of infectious diseases for some years was didactic only, save for the few years in the early '90's when there was an infectious disease department in the hospital. This was closed in 1893. On December 17, 1918, an affiliation with the Alexandra Hospital was arranged([1]) and now each student in the School spends two months in that institution.

([1]) The first students to enter for this training were Miss Hattie Parks and Miss Elsie Sevigny.

CHAPTER X

In this account of the development of the Training School for Nurses events have been allowed to speak for themselves. It will have been obvious that not only the existence of the School but its whole character have been directly dependent on the nature of the hospital from which it has been evolved. It will further be recognized that the lay support and guidance of the hospital and School have been inestimably precious. The generosity and benevolence of attitude of the long line of governors and other benefactors can never be a matter for mere acknowledgment only. They have always been the expression of the purest goodwill, and are so regarded.

As regards the medical aspect of the life of the hospital, however, and its effect on the School, a little more definition is necessary than has been given in the preceding pages.

It will be recalled that when Florence Nightingale established the first training school for nurses, she chose St. Thomas's Hospital for two reasons: the high quality of the medical staff in that hospital, and the outstanding character of its matron. Now, there is no one element of more importance in the history of the Montreal General Hospital than the character of the men on its medical staff. When the institution was first organized its work might well have been carried on with no more than the charity and solicitude to have been expected of physicians. But the founders had another solicitude. They wanted to teach. No other single factor has contributed as much to the standard of work in the hospital as has the medical teaching which has been carried on in it from its very earliest year. Resolution and tenacity of purpose were needed to introduce the idea (indeed, the matter occasioned a duel between Dr. Stephenson and an opponent of the charter); and the carrying out of it has always made severe demands on time and effort. But it is the salt which has helped to preserve very high standards of professional work.

The nurse benefits incalculably from her daily association with these standards. They form an indefinable but none the less valuable element in her training, and they are much more difficult to maintain in the absence of medical teaching.

It is doubtful whether the School for Nurses would have been developed at all if the hospital had not been a medical teaching centre. The first attempt to start the school was undoubtedly due to the efforts on the part of the medical men. The reasons for its failure have already been discussed. Even if the medical men themselves were not entirely blameless in the matter (one of them at least) they did their utmost to carry it on, and lectures for the nurses were kept up fairly steadily during Miss Rimmer's time.

Then came the realization that systematic training had to be instituted, and, after a few weeks of, hesitation (as if it were the fluttering of the wings of destiny), there came Miss Livingston.

The record of Miss Livingston's achievement reads rather breathlessly, so rapid it was, so brilliant, and so sound. But it must not be forgotten that even she might have found it too severe a task for her powers if she had not had the complete support of her medical staff. Most fortunately, she was the right woman for the task, but in the first few years circumstances were so difficult, and mistakes were so easy to make, that she needed all the help she could get, and the medical and administrative staff gave it to her unwaveringly.

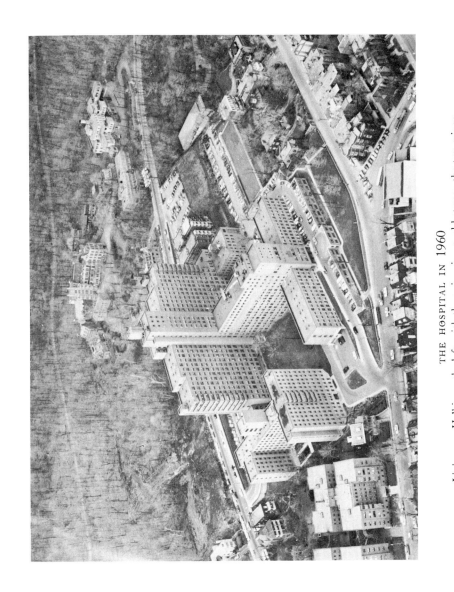

THE HOSPITAL IN 1960

Livingston Hall is on the left, with the swimming pool between the two wings.

CHAPTER XI

The Moving of the Hospital

The two Divisions of the Hospital were transferred to the new site on the slopes of the mountain only six years ago, but in that short time the beneficial consequences have far exceeded even the high expectations with which the move was attended. Indeed, before three years passed the demands on the Hospital became so heavy that considerable additions, both to the Hospital and the nurses' residence, were made, and it is expected that there will be yet others before long.

There had been no definite signs of any such overshadowing project in 1940, unmistakable and urgent as the necessity for expansion was even then becoming; other very different shadows had to be taken into account at that time! However, in 1943 the idea of moving away to a new site, with new buildings, began to be accepted as the solution of the problem, and from then on it became a matter of effort and time. In May, 1948 the site was bought; in May, 1953 the cornerstone of the Hospital was formally laid, and in May, 1954 that of Livingston Hall; in May, 1955 the buildings were occupied for work.

Those seven years have a history of their own. On the administrative side there was the tremendous burden of finance; two successive campaigns for funds were necessary; decisions were made leading to the responsibility for expenditures without precedent in the history of the Hospital. There was the infinitely intricate problem of laying out the buildings, of finding out what each department needed, and of trying to satisfy multiple demands. There were all the additional distractions of a transition period when the work of a busy hospital had to be carried on under steadily contracting circumstances together with rapidly developing commitments a mile away.

In the last six months before the move the mass of preparatory details was yet further (though unintentionally) complicated by the decision of the city to begin widening operations on Dorchester Street in front of the Hospital. In November, 1954 the bulldozers reached the front entrance, and for the first time on record this had to be closed off. At the same time the tunnel beneath the street connecting the Hospital and the Nurses' Home was closed up, and the nurses then had to cross a very busy and often muddy thoroughfare in all weathers.

For two weeks before the move the nursing staff lived in the newly opened Livingston Hall, and were taken to and from work by bus. There may have been some temporary nostalgic memories of the abandoned Nurses Home, for it was a modern building and was very comfortable and well fitted up. Its surroundings, however, were unattractive, if not unsavoury; comment was made in the annual report of 1949 that an increase in applications for training had been noted "in spite of the disadvantages of the district."

But no nostalgia could last long in the face of the sumptuous grandeur of the new Livingston Hall. It has now become familiar but in 1955 the difficulty was to find adjectives to do justice to its splendour, both comparative and actual. And yet, with all its spaciousness and colour it has a happy blending of characteristics which preserve all the warm friendliness of the old residence. It was even arranged to bring up the foundation stone of the old Jubilee Nurses Home, which had been laid by Lord Lister in 1897. It now stands at the side of the Cedar Avenue doorway.

In her address at the laying of the cornerstone of Livingston Hall, as President of the Alumnae Association, Norena Mackenzie said:

" . . . Once again we are renewing our individual and collective responsibility for the School's supreme function—to try to create the best possible conditions for the right development of the young women who enter it.

"We can and ought to speculate about the value of new methods, of curricula, and of the many aspects of an educational programme. But the most important conditions for supplying the demands of growth are the same—yesterday, to-day, and forever. They are the personal qualities and beliefs of those who help to build the School. Poverty at that level cannot be replaced by architecture, equipment, efficiency, or even intellectual brilliance. There must be a 'Vision of Greatness.'

"It is our sincere hope that the trinity of Wisdom, Goodness and Truth will continue to prevail in the School's activities. They are our roots and direction."

High tribute is due to Miss Blanche Herman as Associate Director in charge of Livingston Hall. Miss Herman took over this arduous

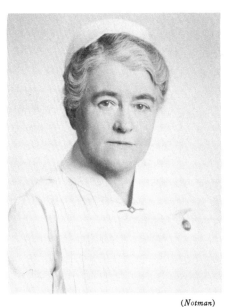

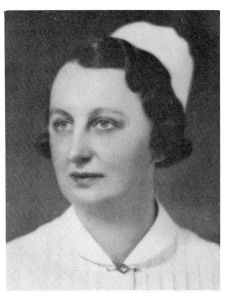

MISS CHRISTINA DENOVAN
Graduated 1920. On Night Staff 1920-23.
Night Superintendent 1932-1955.

MISS BLANCHE HERMAN
Supervisor of Nursing, Western Division.
Associate Director of Nursing in charge of
Livingston Hall.

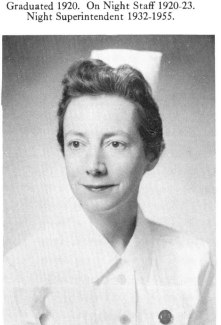

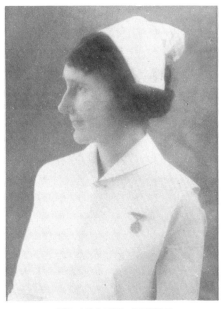

MRS. A. ISOBEL MACLEOD
Director of The School
1961

MISS MARTHA BATSON
Graduated 1921. Post-graduate work at McGill
1924-25. Assistant instructor 1925-27. Educational Director 1928-46. Resigned due to ill
health. Died 1954.

duty after her work at the Western Division terminated. "Every aspect of the life of the residence is her concern, from the smallest fleck of dust to the constant and intricate planning of the frequent receptions and entertainments for which the Hall is so preeminently fitted." (*Alumnae News Letter*, January 1957)

In the Hospital itself the most evident innovation from the nursing point of view was the new type of small unit wards. This had been a deliberate choice, but at first there were some feelings of regret at losing the long, open wards of the Central Division; many congratulatory comments on these had been received from visitors. The new wards also required more staff. However, by the end of 1955 all major changes had been made successfully. If there had been any difficulties to be overcome the patients at any rate were not aware of them.

It is to be remembered that two hospitals were involved in the move, even if they were Divisions of the one institution. The complexity of coordinating the two staffs into one was carried out with complete success. The transfer of the patients was probably the least burdensome part when it was actually carried out, although it called for very careful planning. Some of the wards were gradually emptied beforehand and admissions were cut down, leaving only acute and emergency cases. In the end 70 patients were moved from the Western Division and 105 from the Central. This was done on two successive Sunday mornings (May 22 and 29), to take advantage of favourable traffic conditions: the Western Division was moved first. With splendid police cooperation it was all done in about three hours on each day.

It was quite in keeping with the energy generated by the new hospital atmosphere that in spite of all the pressing readjustments consequent on the move in 1955 the Alumnae Association still found it possible to hold a Reunion in 1956. The planning of this was directed by Mrs. Catherine Townsend,[1] whose unusual abilities and imperturbable good humour were largely responsible for what proved a uniquely successful event, creating the genuine sense of a very large family gathering.

---

[1] Miss Herman had been chairman at first but later found it impossible to meet the combined heavy demands on her time as President of the Alumnae Association and Director of the Hall.

CHAPTER XII

The Changing Curriculum

The education of nurses until not so long ago appeared to be, if not a simple matter, at least one whose demands did not raise much questioning. This was certainly the case during Miss Livingston's regime; her outlook in nursing was a very strong influence for years after her death, indeed, her "the patient must come first" still remains the dominant theme of the School.

Now, however, although that theme is unchanged it has undergone much variation and expansion. The demands on nursing are now so diverse that varying amounts and kinds of preparation are required, calling for increased teaching personnel, which in its turn creates a need for more training of teachers.

The present curriculum definitely reflects the influence of these demands.

The Preliminary Term

There will always be the problem of adjusting the proportionate amounts of theory and practice to be taught in this short period. The basic anatomical and physiological sciences, together with pharmacology and nutrition still take up a large part of the time in this term, but an important change in the nursing training during the last decade has been that the student at the very outset is also introduced to an understanding of the mutual relationships between human beings and their environment.

This is done by means of classes and field trips on Human Growth and Development, and Community Organization. These are designed to bring out the various phases in the entire life of the individual. Observation visits to various centres are made, followed by discussion periods. Here is a beginning at any rate of creating a realization of what chiefly concerns and affects the individual who is the *raison d'être* of the nurse—the patient.

But the basic sciences are still only part of the business of nursing itself, and the major part of the term is spent on basic nursing, through lectures and demonstrations and the all-important bedside teaching; it is here that the main emphasis is placed. The use of dummies in classroom teaching has been considerably reduced. The probationer is taken on a visit to the wards as early as the day after registration, and two weeks later is on the wards daily for two hours for simple nursing procedures.

Along with the increased emphasis on the social sciences there has been a growing attention to training in psychiatric nursing. This is taken up in the intermediate term and is given both at the Hospital itself and at the Verdun Protestant Hospital. It was first introduced in a limited way in 1950, and a two-months period was put into force in 1955, when the full growth of the Psychiatric Department in the Hospital was achieved. The third month is spent at the Verdun Protestant Hospital.

The greater part of the second year is spent on training at "affiliated" hospitals, such as the Montreal Children's Hospital for Paediatrics, and the Alexandra Hospital for six weeks of Communicable Diseases (this is a very long established affiliation). Teaching in the nursing of tuberculosis has been arranged with the Royal Edward Laurentian Hospital, partly at the St. Urbain Street Division, and partly at the Ste. Agathe Division. At the former, two weeks are spent in the Public Health Department visiting in patients' homes; at the latter, the student learns something of the sanatorium treatment of tuberculosis, and through this comes to appreciate some of the problems of long-term illness in general.

The training in obstetrics is still carried on at the Royal Victoria Montreal Maternity Hospital, the lineal descendant of the old Maternity Hospital on St. Urbain Street. But in 1958 this training was first introduced in part into our own obstetric unit. This was achieved after about three years of planning. The affiliation with the R.V.M.M.H. remains as before, and takes care of those students who cannot be absorbed by our own smaller obstetrical unit.

The problem presented by the absence of a prenatal clinic in our Hospital has been met in various ways; the Catherine Booth Maternity Hospital allows students to observe in the prenatal clinic, and gives instruction in other directions; and the Department of Physical Medicine of the Hospital provides for prenatal exercises. It is hoped that eventually it may be possible to arrange for students to participate to some extent in the prenatal and postnatal planning with mothers in their homes, which is so efficiently carried on by the Montreal Branch of the Victorian Order of Nurses.

New subjects have appeared in the curriculum; Group Dynamics; Team Nursing; First Aid and Disaster Nursing. All these reflect the refinements and specialties which arise from modern requirements in nursing. To meet these demands there naturally has been an increase in the number of the staff; there are now ten full time clinical teachers, with Miss Anna Christie as Associate Director of Nursing in charge of Education.

This brief description is in no sense an account of the teaching curriculum. It is only intended to show that there have been changes, and it may be added that these will continue to appear. It is realized that the work of the School must be repeatedly surveyed and critically assessed. In December, 1958, for example, a firm of Management Consultants was requested to make a study of day-by-day activities of the nursing staff. This was to help in determining how the work organization might be changed to use nursing time to the best advantage, and the report submitted gave definite guidance which led to useful alterations in administrative work.

Along with this the School participated in a pilot project for evaluation of Schools of Nursing in Canada; this was shared in by twenty-five schools of nursing, and resulted in a Curriculum Committee being set up in our own School to study methods of teaching.

Post-Graduate Training

As in all progressive schools for professional training the question of post-graduate education was destined to arise eventually. Miss Holt in her annual report of 1939 drew attention to the need to provide further training for those who showed aptitude and desire for post-graduate work.

There are now some scholarships and bursaries in teaching and nursing administration, provided by various groups and by the Hospital itself, to help graduates to take post-graduate courses which have been available at McGill for some years. The vital necessity of post-graduate training in assuring the supply of trained administrators and staff nurses is now so well recognized that a post-graduate course has become a prerequisite in the selection of all teaching and administrative staff.

In the reverse direction an undergraduate course in basic nursing was instituted in the School for Graduate Nurses at McGill in 1957; the Director of our School, Mrs. Isobel MacLeod, is a member of the committee in charge of planning the curriculum. It has been arranged for those taking this course to obtain practical nursing training at this and other city hospitals.

The Second World War

The effects of the second World War on the nursing service in the Hospital were a little less immediate than in 1914, but began to be severely felt by the end of 1940, by which time considerable numbers of graduates were overseas with Canadian hospitals. The number of students, however, continued to be satisfactory; in 1943, for example, there were 198 in the School. The chief effects were in the rapid turnover of staff and the shortage of supplies.

As would be expected, these handicaps were more evident in the Private Patients Pavilion in the Western Division, where graduate nurses were so much in demand. The effects lasted till well after the war. Dr. Lorne Gilday, in charge of the Western Division, and at one period of the war head of both Divisions, noted in his 1948 report: "Nurses come and nurses go, and more seem to go than come." The severe and constant strain to which the Western Division was subjected is clearly reflected in his annual reports.

The Honour Rolls of our Hospital nurses for the two wars are now on the walls of Livingston Hall. The second one was unveiled on March 3, 1958, by Dr. Lorne C. Montgomery, with Mrs. Stuart Ramsey as chairman of the ceremony. Dr. Montgomery from his intimate personal experience of both wars vividly recalled memories of humour, danger and frustration in the military hospital world, as well as of challenge to which there was unfailing response with courage and resourcefulness. The names on these Honour Rolls will be found in Appendix D.

Nursing Assistants

One of the many effects of the war was the shortage of nurses, as already noted. This was variously ascribed to greater demands from industry; the institution of the 8-hour day for graduate nurses; improved economic conditions; and absorption into the Armed Forces. Many nurses at the retiring age came forward to help, but the situation in the early 'forties was extremely acute.

At this stage the nursing assistant became a valuable element in the work of the Hospital. One report (1945) speaks of the Hospital turning more and more to "nursing assistants, practical nurses and trained attendants, not to mention ward helpers."

Under these circumstances, in the fall of 1948 the Montreal School for Nursing Aides began as an experiment, sponsored by five hospitals in the city, including the Montreal General Hospital and the Montreal Convalescent Hospital, where the School first was located. Miss Mary Mathewson, then Director of our Nursing School, was a member of the original committee for its organization.

An extremely useful purpose was served by this School. It was moved to the Reddy Memorial Hospital in 1952, and was finally taken over by the Department of Veterans' Affairs in 1954, to become the Montreal School for Nursing Assistants. It has now been discontinued.

CHAPTER XIII

Nursing in Retrospect

There is one element in the handling of the sick which is not so easy to define or assess, but becomes apparent in comparing nursing now with what it was like forty years ago. This subject was the theme of an address by one of the older alumnae at the extremely successful Reunion in 1956.

The speaker, Miss Margaret J. Denniston spoke on the general theme of bridging the gap between the old and the new Hospitals.

" . . . On one side of the bridge we have left a slower age, a more humane age, with superb service to and interest in the patient as a person. On the other side we have the (unknown) age of rapid change stimulated by scientific discovery and progress. These discoveries have brought many benefits as well as many trials and problems . . . We have to think and act more quickly . . . We emphasize the sociological and psychological aspects of nursing, but have no time to practise either.

"The professional nurse today has to concentrate more on her work than we ever thought of doing, if she or her patient hopes to survive. The nurse, forced to attend to immediate vital needs is frustrated by her inability to find time for the individual human touch. With the introduction of team nursing and early ambulation the bed bath, which is seldom given, has been allocated almost entirely to the nurse aide. The ideal opportunity for the nurse to know her patient a little better and to share her problems has been taken away. For the patient, the nurse is associated with pain—she usually has a needle with her or is not too far away from one.

"No wonder we often hear ex-patients proclaim 'Any nursing I got in hospital was given by the nurse aide.' They are unaware of who is at the helm when the sea is rough during post anaesthesia or when the blood pressure dips to zero."[1]

Miss Denniston really epitomized the heart of the problem in nursing. Nothing recurs more often in writings and comments on modern nursing than the question: Is nursing still as thorough and devoted as it used to be?

---

[1] *Alumnae News Letter:* January 1957.

And yet, intricate as the picture may appear there has been no essential change in the nurse-patient relationship. Certainly the Training School continues to lay steady emphasis on the care of the patient as the central theme. Constant developments there will be and it is in adjustment to these that the School is tested.

Other things than changes in the curriculum must also be considered. One great innovation was the introduction of the 8-hour day. This had been in force for graduate nurses outside the Hospital since 1942, but not until 1953 was it arranged for the Hospital. It is rather impressive to realize that 12-hour duty in the wards had persisted for 60 years; little wonder that it seemed to be a revolutionary change. It brought its problems of arranging for the three tours of duty, but there were no serious difficulties.

A yet further development along the same lines, with the accompanying effects of increasing the numbers of nurses required, as well as all the additional minutiae of administration, has been the initiation of the 5-day week for nursing in the Hospital. This only came into effect on April 1, 1961.

A point of some importance has been the lowering of the admission age of students to 17½ years. Originally, the entrance age had been 21. This was changed to 18 in 1940, and to 17½ in 1958. It had been found that in the interval between school-leaving age and admission to the Nursing School too much potential nursing material was being lost to other occupations. A larger number of applicants for training has resulted, and it has been found advisable to have only one incoming class each year, instead of the customary two. There are now more than 300 girls in training at a time, and in 1957 it was necessary to add two floors to the nurses' residence to accommodate the increased numbers.

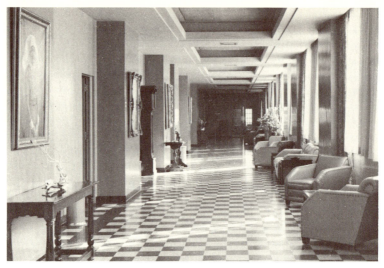

THE SUNNY 'PEACOCK ALLEY' IN LIVINGSTON HALL

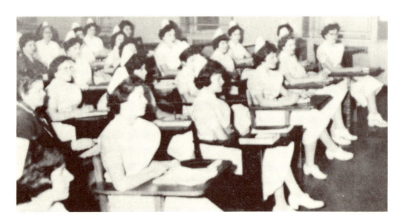

A FINAL YEAR CLASS

The graduation age is lower than when The School began. Compare these students in their third year with the graduating classes in Miss Livingston's regime.

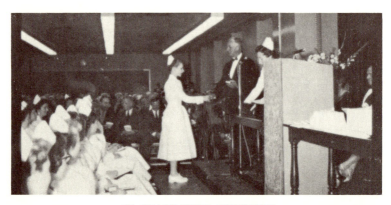

AT GRADUATION CEREMONY

CHAPTER XIV

The Mentor Programme

The size of the School itself presents certain problems which did not exist in its earlier years. As has been shown, a class is registered each year, in September, and this numbers about 120. This means that at any one time there are more than 300 students in the School, and it has been well recognized that in such a large group, drawn from such diverse sources, there may be in some at least a feeling, if not of being lost, at any rate of wanting to feel at home.

It was with the idea of combating this aspect of bigness that in 1959 the Mentor programme was initiated. Its object in the main is that of providing personal support for each student through the counsel and interest of staff members chosen as mentors. Four students are assigned to each mentor, and a regular scheme of keeping in touch has been arranged throughout the whole course, with somewhat longer intervals as the course proceeds.

Not only does the student benefit directly from this close contact with sympathetic guidance, but the mentors themselves by pooling their experience in regular meetings amongst themselves, are able to understand some of the factors underlying both failure and success amongst the students. They are thus able to forestall avoidable causes of failure, especially in the first year, or to offer suggestions about them, as well as to gain insight into the characteristics common to those who succeed in their course. Valuable comment on the criteria for selecting future students may develop as a result of this experience.

Nursing Associates

Yet another group activity associated with the students is the formation of the M.G.H. School of Nursing Associates, which also came into being in 1959. This organization is composed of parents or guardians of students. Its general aim is to serve as a channel for keeping its members and the general public informed about the objectives of the School, thus providing a better understanding of the nursing profession and promoting the interests of the School. It also aids in obtaining bursary assistance for needy students.

This organization is still in process of finding itself, but there has been enough interest in it already to lead to considerable activity both practical and social.

The Staff Nurses Association

This Association has been in existence since 1957. Its membership is solely amongst the non-administrative nurses. Its object is to promote a spirit of unity and a common bond of understanding and mutual helpfulness among the staff nurses of the Hospital. It also has the function of providing an organization which can speak officially for the staff, in presenting their views on problems arising in the work of nursing in the Hospital.

Transient Nurses

The mobility of the staff constitutes a constant problem. It is interesting and gratifying that the School should attract nurses of every nationality, but a great many of these move on after only a comparatively short stay. They are obeying the restlessness of our period, to which the ease and speed of travel contribute so markedly, not to mention the certainty of finding nursing employment in so many countries.

It is natural that such a constant and quickly changing stream of those who in the main are little more than visitors, should produce problems in maintaining the esprit de corps which has always been so strong in the School. One method of improving the situation has been a definite programme of orientation for new nurses coming to work in the Hospital. This means that in the first week arrangements are made for the detailed introduction of the nurse to all departments of the Hospital, together with periods for discussing professional, cultural, and entertainment opportunities in Montreal. A carefully prepared programme covering all these points is given to each nurse on reporting to the Hospital.

The Women's Auxiliary

The work of the Women's Auxiliary has become so closely—and pleasantly—bound up with the life of the Hospital and Nursing School that some reference, brief only as it can be here, must be made to its growth.

It has been well said by Mrs. Burnett Johnston that the Women's Auxiliary has really recaptured the spirit of the devoted women of Montreal through whose efforts in 1817 to help the sick poor the House of Recovery came into being, the seed from which grew the Montreal General Hospital.

There was then no thought of an Auxiliary; various gifts used to flow into the Hospital, especially at Christmas, as the expression of charitable impulses, but it was very long before these came to have any organized direction. However, in 1949 there came about what was called "the fortunate coincidence when interested women of Montreal expressed their willingness to organize an Auxiliary, and at the same time the Hospital realized the need of the services offered."

That was how Mrs. Alexander Hutchison, the first President of the Auxiliary, described its beginnings, but it would not be wrong to suppose that it was from the "interested women" that there came the all-important initial impulse which brought about such an achievement.

Its title really falls far short of indicating the intimately permeating influence of the Auxiliary. With the aim of providing to patients and the staff services which gratefully complement what can be expected of the Hospital, the Auxiliary has taken the fullest advantage of its opportunities. The thought behind what it can do for the patient opens up channels of beneficence in many directions. For the School of Nursing it contributes funds to help student nurses in completing their training; it took on the responsibility for the interior adornment of Livingston Hall; it has donated equipment and furnishings of the most varied nature; and it has created an atmosphere of goodwill and desire to help which attracts many graduates into its membership.

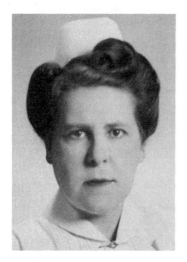

MISS MARY MATHEWSON
Director of The School 1945-1953

Mary Seabury Mathewson was born in Montreal on June 25th, 1898.

A graduate of the School for Nursing in 1925 Mary Mathewson early showed evidence of the absorption in her profession which, with her outstanding qualities of mind and personality made her an immediate choice as Director of the School on the retirement of Miss Holt in 1945. Her qualities of administration had been well tested as Assistant Director of the McGill School for Graduate Nurses.

Miss Mathewson came to her main life's work at a time when the physical circumstances of the Hospital were fast reaching the stage of inadequacy which was to lead eventually to the building of an entirely new hospital. Unhappily, she was destined to witness only the early planning. Her lot was to guide the School through the difficult post-war years, in their disruptive atmosphere, and in the face of a steadily rising pressure of demands on the Hospital. Her equable temperament and determination were exactly suited to dealing with these conditions; she neither shirked nor complained. She died on March 13, 1953, too soon to see the transformation of the School, but she died at her work, which is as she would have had it.

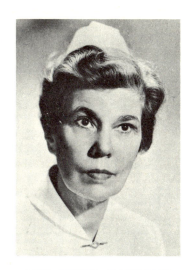

MISS NORENA MACKENZIE

Norena Mackenzie was born in Teeswater, Ont. on June 14, 1899. After graduation in the School of Nursing in 1926 she took a year of post-graduate study at the School of Graduate Nurses at McGill in 1928. As assistant instructor at her Alma Mater School (1929-30) her unusual teaching powers were fully recognized, and in 1932 she was chosen at an International Council of Nurses' meeting in Montreal as one of two Canadian nurses, to study nursing in Great Britain under the Florence Nightingale Fund.

After various overseas appointments during and after the war she became Director of Nursing Education at the M.G.H. in 1947 and held this position for eight years. In 1951 she was appointed a nursing consultant to the World Health Organization, and later was called to a meeting of the Expert Commission on Nursing, in Geneva. In 1955 she accepted the Educational Directorship of the School for Nurses at the Jewish General Hospital. In the fall of 1958 her health failed and she died on January 13, 1959.

APPENDIX A

MISS LIVINGSTON'S LETTERS

[The following extracts are from some of Miss Livingston's letters to her two sisters, Gracie and Alice, who at the time (1890-91) were travelling on the Continent. The originals contain a great deal of personal material which cannot be published, but it was felt that what is given here has interest not only as a sidelight on Miss Livingston herself, but as a commentary on people and conditions in the hospital. Her reflections were made of course with no idea of their being made public, and due care has been exercised in making the selections.]

June 18, 1890.

Dear Alice: Just got your letter. Now about my dresses. I have got nothing since you left. My grey has not been touched. I will have it done in March before the rush of work . . . . It is something awful how dresses wear out when you wear them from morning till night. Miss S. is sending me a little sewing girl—75c a day—who can make me a dress such as my brown. Miss O'Dowd is something awful—such a fitting skirt, and the sleeves I can put both hands in. But it is the same with everything here. No skilled workers—and the concerts! Why, it is a perfect farce. One misses the lack of public entertainment—and if anything does come it creates as much stir as a man at a tea fight. I tell you the Americans are away ahead in every way.

I will deposit $25 as soon as I get my pay. I could not do it sooner last month for we were not paid till the 7th—some red tape nonsense. . . . . We have been very busy—Dr. K.([1]) sick, which complicates things . . . and such a time as I have had with that bad girl Nurse Green, but she was sent away on Saturday for good. You remember my laying the cake trap for her. Well, she did not rise to that fly, but the other night Nurse Darling found a silk photo frame gone. So I said I would start and search the rooms. . . . There is no doubt that she is the guilty party—so young and lovely—how sad. It turns out now that she is not 18. (There was later proof of this nurse having stolen a diamond ring, and Miss

---

([1]) Dr. Kirkpatrick, the medical superintendent.

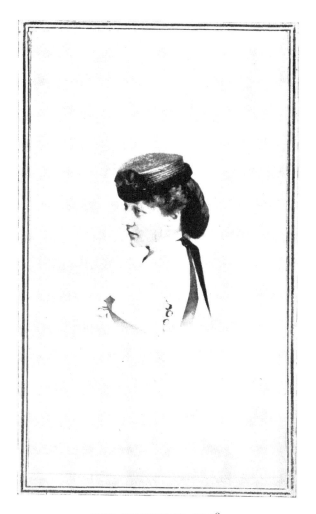

MISS LIVINGSTON AT 18

Livingston continues:) I could have had her arrested, and she could have got two years in the penitentiary, but it would have ruined the school.

June 29, 1890.

. . . Those beastly reporters—they get hold of everything· They came here but we said we had nothing to say. But everybody in Montreal does their work so badly, and of course the "kitchen" had to talk, but it cannot be helped, and it is over now.

I am busy. Monday, Tuesday and Wednesday, class nights, and Saturday lecture, but I feel well and am growing thinner. Our typhoid nurse very ill. Such a sweet girl; was a very light case at first, but she had a relapse and it is very bad. I am afraid of perforation, but I hope for the best. I dread a nurse dying, but I hope it will not come to that. Frank([1]) has just told me that Mrs. Savage is not expected to live, and Annie Gault has been operated on—"vermiform appendix".

Miss Quaife([2]) still goes out with Mr. McIver. He sends her Ruskin to read. It is amusing too. He certainly is doing well. Her influence over him is good. But to see Mrs. G.,([3]) who is the most curious woman. There is really nothing she will not ask— perfectly tactless. She cannot afford to get books that she enjoys, and to see Q. in the throes of Ruskin and Drummond *urges* G. It would work up well in a book.

The way I have to manage all these people! I could hang them all round. The other day a nurse was sick—it was suspected typhoid. Dr. K. saw her, and said milk diet till Dr. McDonnell saw her. Miss Quaife quietly put on poultices and gave her tea and toast. Dr. K. was furious—said he would report her to the medical board—that she was too officious—could not mind her own business. I smoothed him down. He says Quaife is too well paid, and has not the breeding to know a lady when she sees one. That is quite true. At the same time it serves my purpose to keep her. You know she has a way of waiting till Dr. K. goes out, and then says "I'll go for McKechnie", which I never allow. The other day she attempted it. I heard her asking Dr. McK. to see a ward maid who was sick, and I knew Dr. K. was in, but Dr. McK., just as I was going to speak, said, "Where is Kirk? I am very particular as to professional etiquette." Besides, they are great friends, and it is an irregular thing.

My floor is to be laid soon, and it will be very nice. I have nothing to do with anything which is not . . .

([1]) Dr. F. J. Shepherd.
([2]) Her assistant.
([3]) Mrs. Greatorex, the night superintendent.

I do not think Canadians are worth a rush for punch. If they sneeze—off to bed. We have seven employees laid up now—colds and nonsense. They are so punchless. Of course I am down on the milk we get here. I think our nurses never get typhoid from the patients. I made a fuss and it was analyzed, but Mr. Bates went down to the "farm" at Longue Pointe on Sunday, and he says it looks dirty. Penny wise and pound foolish. For one cent we suffer. I never touch milk. I am well and happy, but oh, so busy.

November 23, 1890.

Professor Penhallow([1]) called on me yesterday—very Yankee . . . The little boy came with them and gave me some toys for the children's ward.

Bella is quite sick so I have Matilda for my rooms. Really I cannot understand what Lily([2]) meant about her work. You would think she had lived with the bears—the table half set—I had to tell her over and over again what to do. Matilda is such a comfort and so clean. Bella would forget morning after morning to dust and empty the waste basket—in fact, she made me mad. She was like a dream. Dr. Molson says her heart is affected—I should say it was her brain.

The Committee are pondering about plans, etc. I hope they will not build, as they really have not the money to support and run the pavilions after they are built. Miss Nilson goes tomorrow. She has become quite lively here. She is coming to the Training School in Feb. (fad of Frank's)—one week of 31 will decide her vocation.

There has been quite a panic in the Stock Market, but it is all over, and now stocks are lower. C. Pacific was the stock which fell. I got my receipts and policy today, so that is satisfactorily settled—and I am paying my debts, then I will start fresh—and I am well equipped—I wish I was a nun: no bother as to fal lals! !

November 29, 1890.

The weather very cold—no snow. I got a letter yesterday from Miss Snively, Toronto Hospital, asking me what I got here as salary, and saying that St. Luke's gives $1,500, Johns H[opkins] the same. But Dr. McDonnell coming in at the time I told him, and asked him if he thought I could ask $1,000. He said, *No*, as he said "Cows at a distance have long horns" . . . Miss S. would no doubt use my letter if suitable to ask for an increase

---

([1]) Professor of Botany at McGill University. It is possible that he was responsible for the planting along the hospital fence on Lagauchetiere and St. Dominique Streets of the three fine gingko trees—the Japanese sacred tree.

([2]) Mrs. F. J. Shepherd.

from her hospital. But I am too canny—I will just give her facts. Anyone can see my salary from the reports.

January 5, 1891.

. . . I have heard that Dr. Craik has had $5,000 given to him for the hospital. It is to be specially announced. That is what the opening([1]) did for us. It was certainly worth the expenditure of $50.00, and just fancy, the Committee are going to give gold medals—nearly the size of ours.

Everything is going on nicely here. Miss Q. goes out with Mr. McI. and I do not mind, for she is old enough to judge for herself. Of course there is nothing in it. She told me that she will gladly remain as long as the Committee will keep her. I fancy she knows that the . . . are not going to leave her any money.

. . . By the way, I must tell you that yesterday I was down in Ward 11, and luckily happened to be standing at the window looking into my rooms, when to my astonishment I saw my gas centre seemingly on fire. I flew down the hall and on my way picked up one of the pails of water, and found that Bella in lighting the gas had lit up the green decorations—and the whole thing in a blaze and she standing open-mouthed doing nothing. I put out the gas and fire. Nothing the worse, but I think I will insure my clothes and piano for $1,000. I would feel both mad and sad if anything happened—the doctors have their things insured.

I will go up later to Como. I cannot leave here—two nurses sick—Miss Hall gone home, sore feet, but is getting better. Nurse Haggart, we are afraid, has typhoid fever—a light case. Canadians do not seem to have any grit. I would rather have that quality than any other in a nurse; it pulls them through when all else gives out.

The House Committee came in yesterday with the medal designs—quite realistic, but well designed—gold. They are to be about the size of mine. There is a pretty little sketch of a nurse in our uniform standing by a hospital bed. I put the old "pap spoons" up to gold instead of silver, by taking it for granted that *we* could not *afford* gold. They will come to about $10.00 apiece after the die is bought. He gave out invitations (for the opening) by card. We have the whole thing in magazine form. Dr. Craik added the little tribute to Miss Q. and after all one must remember not to be jealous and narrow about her being mentioned. She has done well, and I know her thoroughly—good points and bad. But she is a great comfort to me, and after all, like all Americans, she is no fool about Mr. McI. They know how to take care of themselves —at least she does.

([1]) The graduation ceremonies for the second graduating class.

Just fancy—Dr. — has given me $100 for my floor. Now I have $267 and will start on bedsteads.

January 24, 1891.

. . . It amuses me your saying you would be full of vanity if you were me. I can tell you who would be and that would be Quaife. She hates to hear me praised, and she is not well enough bred to hide it. Now we are the best of friends, but I can see through her. Dr. K. sits on her about her jealousy of me. Dr. K. gave me a beautifully bound copy of the "Opening"—and it was very kind of him, but after all anyone in his position would have done the same—it would naturally suggest itself, but Q. would not even notice it, and of course Mrs. G. exclaimed at its being so nice of him to give it, and how pretty it was, etc.

I got a letter from Mrs. Gibb asking for a nurse, as old Ann is very ill—but the requirements! She must be competent, trustworthy, willing to eat with the servants—sleep in Ann's room, etc. Now I have just such a "being", but I have to use her here in the "Dr." ward. She was a probationer but would not do for the school, but her story is a sad one, and I keep her for emergencies and to supplement. She is as good as gold, but the hospital must come first. . . . What a busy life this is. The days fly by. It seems but yesterday that I came—a year on the 22nd of February.

February 3, 1891.

. . . I know my last letters were short but one has so little that is amusing. . . . About Mr. McI.—he only comes to take Q. out, is never in to spend an evening. You know he is such a nice man—highly educated—up in everything. Gave Q. "Sesame & Lilies" and some of Drummond's latest. She wrestles with them!!! He sent me a copy of "Apologia pro vita sua" (J. H. Newman). You know he is not young—about 50 I should say—very gentlemanly—but Q. is cute and enjoys being taken about by him. But she is very discrete. I well know people would say it was me he came to see if he spent the evening.

Now that it's all over I must tell you of my little breeze with the Committee. You remember my telling you Dr.— gave me $100 towards the "Floor Fund". He telephoned the message—said it was deposited with the Treasurer, Mr. W. F. Thomas. So, knowing that Dr. — is not always *quite straight* I telephoned to Mr. T. with whom the money had been lodged. He would not consider it as a gift for the Fund, (though) Dr. — said it was. So, after all this kow towing I gave my $157 to Mr. Thomas and then made a requisition for a new floor, which I am to get. But in future the Committee wish me to deposit all sums given me with Mr. T. and then make a requisition for what I may want.

Dr. K. told me what they were going to do, so I wrote a nice little note saying that in keeping money "in trust" I erred through ignorance, and had no desire to thwart in any way the authority of the committee. The floor is to be of maple, two inches wide. But I am not to have a side border. After all, it is better to give in gracefully when one knows one has to, but I did feel mad and indignant that I would not have what I had collected the money for. Luckily they sent Mr. Alexander to interview me, and he is so old and not at all lucid. So I did not say what I might. However, as Dr. McD. says, eat a little humble pie, for you got your own way in the main. In future I will find out what I want and *someone will present the article*. It quite put me out at the time, but it has all blown over now and we are all good friends.

. . . Young Mr. Larkin who was a "private patient" and a nephew of Mrs. Savage's was telling me about her death. He sometimes comes down in the evening—nice boy, in the bank.

Mrs. T. is very gossipy. They say that the fast young married clique do nothing but gamble, and for big sums. Poker is the game, and Mrs. T. added, "I could believe anything of a woman who would play poker"—it made me laugh. Dr. McDonnell comes in of an evening and we play for matches—very harmless dissipation. But people here are all so narrow. It is decided that he will not be med. supt. I am sorry, but he is going to be married, and of course it would not do—bad combination, and would make complications. That is an important factor in our management who the med. supt. is. Why Dr. Kirkpatrick can't stay put is too provoking, because we get on so well together.

It amuses me to hear about the good clothes. If I have not heard enough about my appearance—you would fancy I wore a fig leaf in common. Quaife, who thinks she has such taste, does not like it. We were laughing the other day about something we wanted, and Dr. K. says, "If Miss Livingston will put on that lovely dress and bonnet and ask for it, it is ours." Poor Q. foams. . .

I hear Dr. Smith is going to apply for med. supt. Well, he is sober and fairly nice, but not much tact. But I have nearly everything in my own hands now—keep all the supplies. You see, Dr. K. lets me give them out—and so, Dr. Smith, if elected, takes things as he finds them. Dr. K. could just as well stay. But he will be back again after a year's experience. He is so easy to work with—good and considerate for me—and he knows Quaife. He said last night— "Oh, she shows the cloven hoof". She must have slanged me last summer pretty well—but those people always defeat themselves. You must not think because I tell you all this, that we do not agree. We get along beautifully, but I never let her take an inch. Dr. K. tells me not to trust her.

Had another nice visit from Dr. McDonnell today. How nice he is. What good manners! The other day I came out just as he was getting out of his sleigh. He said, "Where are you going?" and I said, "To Mrs. Shepherd's"—so he sent me up in his sleigh—so thoughtful.

. . . Really, Mrs. H. ought to be spanked, and soundly too. She that was brought up in a two-inch hole to talk about travel. "Her dead darling" never made her send the $100 for the "Floor Fund". She talks a lot of *rot*.

. . . Just three years since I went to the New York Hospital. I have earned $1,250 in that time.

February 8, 1891.

We have had quite a busy day. Sad death in the private ward. P. Duggan's father—such a nice patient. It was a case of "extirpation of the tongue", and when we thought him out of danger hæmorrhage set in and he died almost at once. They are such decent, respectable people. Nurse Haggart is still very ill, but I think out of danger. I have never yet despaired of her, for I know how bad a typhoid can be and yet live.

I had a long visit from Agnes[1] today. I think she will make up her mind to leave Miss Rimmer—it is a case of dividends payable above, and Agnes evidently does not like the security. . . . It would be lovely to have her back again, but it is all in the dim future as yet. Frank puts up with a lot of bullying from Miss R. for the sake of the people whom she knows.

Miss Q. is going to the theatre with the "reformed one". She bought herself a beautiful cloak—loose—$47.00. By the way, I wish you would see what one of those wraps is in Paris. They are most useful.

I have had such a beauty probationer in. I say "have", because when she is able she is going. You can conceive nothing more lovely—fair—such hair. She, after two days' duty asked if I minded if she came on late in the morning!!! She is a niece of a splendid nurse, and she laughingly said "I thought she would sicken of it, and she is well off and has a comfortable home." Come to find out, it is the rebound from a love affair. . . . The funny ideas that some women have of hospital nursing life is rich—more poetical than practical. After all, it is half the best which do not sift out.

Another one stayed two days, and on coming down to say good-bye said: "To think that you commenced that way—it seems impossible!!"

February 17, 1891.

I had permission from the Committee (to go to Como) and I intended going Thursday when Drs. Vidal and Hamilton[2] wanted

---

[1] Miss Rimmer's maid.
[2] Dr. H. D. Hamilton.

me to give a five o'clock tea to their lady friends, and asked me to entertain and receive for them. So I concluded to do the thing I did not like, which meant the thing I ought, a la Pellico. I am going to give them my sitting-room and fix it up. They know nice people both of them, and for the sake of the hospital I want it nice. They were going to use Dr. McKechnie's room!!! Bed so in corner (a sketch) and everything to match—primeval loveliness.

You ask me if I go out—yes, every day, just for a little spin. Both Q. and I find we must . . . Do not fret about the "contagious wards". Why, I am acclimatized to bad smells and contagion.

Frank laughingly said yesterday that you wanted Lily to go over. I think she could not stand the crossing. He would let her go if I would take her! I wonder what old "pap spoons" would say did I ask a leave of absence, expenses paid!!!

I am glad Alice thinks my writing has improved—it is, I have no doubt, more legible.(¹) . . . How nice it will be to see you again. I have not time to think of how far away you are, but if you were here I could see so much of you. So nice to have you for dinner and tea and in that respect I can "do just as I have a mind to" as Miss Quaife would say.

Did I tell you that little A. gave up a class; sprained her ankle wearing a Cinderella shoe. By the way, Bella M. is married to Dr. C. and old mother M. is pleased at last—"Me daughter has fulfilled her destiny". We are all surprised at it, for Dr. C. was not the soul of honour.

Now, to give you an idea of yesterday. Busy all morning, and Mr. G.—governor—came in. Then Miss Brown, Mrs. King, Mrs. Borelle, Mrs. Drysdale, the last on good works. I got out of her a little flannel gown for the children's ward. Then I just settled down when Nurse McKay felt sick and came down to see me—then Dr. K. had to see her, and before she was done Bella appeared with sore feet, which had to be seen to. Before Dr. K. left it was time for dinner. Then class, and then I went for a walk with Mrs. Greatorex—and so it is every day.

February 20, 1891.

. . . How I hate to think of all the doctors going away. If Dr. K. was not leaving it would not be so bad. Still,"Bates"(²) is the only one in the house whose place cannot be supplied. He is invaluable. Dr. K. I believe would stay if I urged him, but it would hardly be fair to him. Dr. Evans will, I think, get the position, he is so well known socially. I think I will get my summer dress at Carsley's.

(¹) Not much more! [Ed.].
(²) The steward.

. . . Well, our party is over—it was a great success. I think I have a fine head for entertaining. My room looked lovely. I had my big centre table put in my bedroom. It was set up so as to be seen from my sitting-room. We had ice cream, water ices, claret-cup, cake and tea. Mrs. Hamilton lent us a dozen silver spoons and d'oyleys, and the Drs. rented claret cups.

There were about 25 altogether. Nice girls. One pretty girl, a Miss Elliott, sister married to one of the Drs. . . . There were Drs. Evans, Vidal and Hamilton, Dr. K. and Mr. Larkin. It was very nice. I wore my blue (new) cap and white spotted fichu—Miss Q. her uniform, for she had to be in and out of the room to the wards. Dr. K. lent me his plants—they were all abloom, or growing.

. . . I had a letter today from Lady Stanley. The hospital is finished—holds about 40 beds—and she has asked me to find her a Lady Supt., salary $500, with promise of increase. I think between ourselves she thought I might possibly like to go. Such a nice letter. She says "We shall want someone with a great deal of tact because she will have to educate people here to the idea of trained nurses, and she must make her reforms carefully so as to offend none. She must be a Canadian".

I am tired tonight, for after the "party" we had dinner and Dr. Major gave a long lecture. He is very nice, but has changed from the good-looking young man I remember . . . I think from what I hear that Dr. Evans will be the next med. supt. Well, since we can't keep Dr. K. he is next best, for he is a gentleman and has nice friends, and a nice way to work with. Perhaps I may sing another tale this time next year. I am beginning to trust no one, not even myself.

Oh, Quaife would like Ottawa. She is jealous. I have so much in my power. Still, you must remember that though I tell you all these little "behind the scenes" she is a good faithful worker and I have no trouble with her, for she has a firm grip as far as she can go. Often of a Sunday morning she brings me my breakfast in bed just as I am going to get up. She has good sense in many things and is not a stupe(?) like Mrs. Greatorex. No pushing her to her work. So she has good qualities, barring her jealousy.

Our medal is to be hospital on one side—very pretty and more dignified than the nurse. The latter was too personal. Dr. Craik allowed me to put it to the vote among the nurses and all chose the hospital. After all, as I said, they earn and wear it—they may be consulted.

The sewing here is not what it was. I would pack Margaret off—she suits herself in the time she gives. Really, Mrs. Gibb works hard—makes all the bread, etc.—Ann in her room, useless—little Mary working like a beaver. I consider M. an ungrateful woman to so neglect her work and employees. She looks like an old dog, but does (not) behave like one. Mrs. Cully and Minnie G.

said Mrs. G. should get some capable woman, for now if ever, they both need care. But they do both look so well and bright. What wonderful people.

. . . I am going out with Mrs. G. for a drive this afternoon. I shall be glad to get back to the hospital. I am very happy here. I wonder could I ever live out of that atmosphere of bells, patients and bad smells. Miss Q. is just as pleased to be there as I am. She seems to have forgotten all about New York. Certainly it is not its beauty. But the Drs. are just the same. Won't they miss it when they go out as licensed assassins.

Koch's lymph(¹) is as Frank says, all rot. Most certainly they have killed one dear child with it. Of course the parents were willing to try the experiment, but she was such a dear little thing.

March 4, 1891.

I am sorry that you should be so troubled about Dr. Mc-Donnell's coming in *alone* and showing Mrs. G. and myself and Q. how to play poker for about half an hour. I must have written a glowing description if you take such a dissipated view of the matter. He called once again and then it dropped. Dr. K. never spent an evening in my sitting room. And you are not just, for you say "They are not my equals". Why, this staff are all gentlemanly fellows—go out everywhere—lots of nice friends—and I know Miss Q. better than you can, and she does not intimidate me. Nor has she any hold over me. She is a good faithful worker. She is jealous of me because she hears me praised—which is very injudicious of the people who praise me.

I do not wish to imitate any Superintendent—Miss Rimmer, who had a "staffery" once a week—Miss Machin who fell in love with a boy—nor Miss Sutcliffe(²), who used to go to Miss Frank's room and play whist with the staff. It was not considered so bad. But, mind you, I do not bring these instances forward to follow their example. For you are right—*I hate cards*. I knew in this little place people might talk.

Miss Quaife is away in New York. She was sick. Dr. Mc-Donnell said she must go away for a change. She was just run down. She will be back probably in a couple of weeks . . . . Of course I miss her for she does not run to me with every little worry and whim, and she knew her place, for I am very open with her. I say I want it done so—that is my way, and I have the right to order. She is in a proper state of subjection. Dr. K. is as unreasonable in regard to her as you are. I know her faults and her good points. She is not all bad, as you would believe. I can see through Miss Quaife and so can everyone. She is not close enough to hide

(¹) Tuberculin used for treatment.
(²) In another hospital.

95

what she feels. Of course she would like my position, but as long as Dr. K. is above ground she will never get over it. She has been rude to him because he makes nothing of her and defers to me in everything, as he should. She belongs to the class that "keeps company" but even he sees what you not being with her cannot see —that her manner, speech, education, preclude her from any position where such would be required.

My floor is a failure—badly laid. The committee have behaved shamefully—took my money and old Alexander made a mess of it. Mr. T. was in this morning and spoke very angrily about the matter and Mr. Garth considers it a disgrace. He says if he was on the House Committee he would not accept it. The Medical Board are furious. I spoke to the contractor too. I told him I would rather have him take it away than have it.

Really, people are very trying. But by this time next week I will be enthusiastic over bedsteads. I do not pin my faith to any of them, but the wards must look nicely even if the committee are ashamed of themselves, which they are over this floor business.

March 5, 1891.

We are in the depths of March snow. . . . Mrs. S. is coming for me to drive to see the "birdcage"—Church Home. . . . Do not fret about me. I am prim as usual.

March 8, 1891, Sunday afternoon.

Very busy day, notwithstanding it was Sunday. Frank sent word he would operate—emergency case. I got everything ready, Alicia being out, and then when he came down changed his mind. Then Dr. Roddick is coming down this afternoon—another emergency, but Alicia is on hand. The nurses are all so very nice to me. I can get them to do anything. Of course they *would have* to, but it is much pleasanter to have "willing service".

Sunday evening—had to leave off here, and now it is eight o'clock and I will be going to bed soon. How the time does fly.

Miss Quaife will be back on Wednesday. She needed the change, but Dr. McDonnell thinks she lacked pluck, but after all one is only human, and everyone is not blessed with an iron constitution like mine. No earthly compensation can make up for health. I am feeling better than I did in the autumn. My stiff knees (hysterical knees as Grace would call them) are quite well.

. . . Had quite a visit from Frank today. Poor fellow, he makes me sorry. Such a houseful of sick people—it is so discouraging. . . . But Dorothy is so sweet. She is very anxious to know how old her mother is—and Lily said, "Well, about 30", and she answered "Oh, now I don't want any abouts".

We had such a sad case in the children's ward. A little French girl—"Koch's treatment" has done for her—and she is so sweet and pitiful. The faculty are afraid of it now—it is quite a failure, and very wisely have stopped giving it. There is *no cure* on record.

The pavilions will be roofed in by next Fall. All the stone for the foundations is drawn. They are to be of brick, and what a fine "operating-room". Do I bore you with all the hospital chit-chat? I hope not, but I want you to feel how happy I am in my work. I think this has been the happiest year in my life, for I have got where I wanted to be and everything has gone well. Mrs. Simpson was nice to me and I value praise which she gives. She said, "Well, Miss Livingston, Montreal ought to be proud of you and your work".

You know, it seems a tremendous undertaking to outsiders, but it really has not been. I hope the new staff will work all right. I have this one properly trained. Dr. K. has been kind and good to me, kind and considerate in every way. I shall miss him, for he never flirts with the nurses. I hope Dr. Evans will be the same. When Dr. E. came and asked me if I would recommend him to the Board and Mr. T. Davidson I had a pretty plain talk with him. He is a nice fellow. Mr. Davidson said to him that he would vote as Miss Livingston wished.

My nurses are to be examined by Dr. Roddick and Dr. Mc-Donnell. I will be glad when it is all over and they are gone. They have done well and are good nurses, but the old training clings to them like a leach.

March 15, 1891.

. . . The hospital is very light—never been so since I have been here. I suppose it is the examinations going on makes it so. This is the last week. Dr. Bell sails for Berlin tomorrow and Frank comes on as attending. I miss Dr. B. I quite like him, and Frank is so inconsiderate and so much fuss and feather, but good in the main. I went up to Lily's yesterday afternoon, and Frank made me go over with him to the loan exhibition at the Art Rooms. Pretty good, but oh, Canadians are so slow—so way back—so provincial.

I am glad you know some artists. I was glad you went to the "At Home" at the W.'s. My eye, what lots you bought for $9.00. I will send you $10.00 to expend for me as you think best.

The nurses go out on April 1. Dr. Roddick and Dr. McD. examined them. I will have no exercises, but they will have a dance in the evening. I am not sorry they are going. . . . We are anxious as to the new staff, but Dr. McD. told me the other day that if I had any trouble with any of the doctors to come to him. He is so nice, and you may trust him. Dr. Evans will get the appointment as med. supt.

How early the flowers must be in Paris, and how cheap. I nearly always have flowers in my room. Yesterday Mrs. Girdwood called and left me some lovely roses. I should like to know her.

Dr. Girdwood was in the hospital with a bad case—C.P.R.—he saw me and asked me who I was, so that is how she called.

I must tell you that Nurse Sinclair's sister took sick and nurse asked for leave to go and see her, and on going stayed. Then the case being a serious one she was removed to Dr. Gardner's. Then I wrote to her and said that she must now report for duty. So long as her sister depended on her for care I allowed her to stay, but at Dr. G.'s hospital she would not be needed, and that if she wished to resign I was willing, but she was to decide and at once, what she was going to do, for her absence was neither fair to her fellow-nurses or to the hospital.

I spoke to Dr. Roddick about it, for you know the mother has a tongue, and he said just send the note and I will back you, and yesterday he told me that he had a conversation with my little nurse, and that she would return, and sure enough she appeared—and so "discipline was maintained". Dr. Gardner also told me that he wished her to return as he had no use for her. It was nice of them both to back me up, was it not? . . .

I was interested in what you told me about the lack of trained nurses in Paris. Do not the sisters nurse them? How I should like to visit the hospitals abroad. I wonder if I ever will. I expect not. Well, the hospital is the same everywhere—one cannot be more than among sick people.

The "Children's Ward" is such a comfort to me. Such sweet things as we have in it now. Agnes no more scowls—getting quite better. Puts up her little finger at me and says—"Lady, me go home tomorrow". Bad floor as it is, it looks beautiful.

I am anxious to hear what you think of my little photo. Frank makes great fun of it. He asked me if there was not a halo round Santa Nora's head. But Lily laughs and says "Frank thinks you just as nice as I do".

The lectures for the nurses are coming to a close. No more after April or rather March 22. Dr. McDonnell was too tired last night to come down. So, Dr. K. lectured instead. I am sorry he is going for I have trained him down to a *very fine* point. I think the Committee are making a mistake not to try and keep him, for he knows the running, and with me to run him we go on smoothly. He is stubborn enough, but I can manage him, and he is always gentlemanly.

March 19, 1891.

. . . I had a visit from such a nice nurse—supt. of a hospital in Concord, N.H., a Canadian—beautifully dressed. How I wish I was thin and tall—one looks so nicely—it is so much easier to look well in any clothes.

. . . It is very cold again, quite like winter. . . . Frank is busy with the exams. but he is an inconsiderate man, and really he only makes me laugh. He gets in such a stew over his students...

It seems I have so little to tell you this week. A Miss Tippet from the Mass. Gen. Hospital has been to see me in regard to the Supt.'s position in Ottawa. So I told her to write direct to Ottawa and not through me—very much more business-like and official.

Have just come in—was up to Mrs O. about my grey dress. It will be a nice spring dress for me. Miss Sutton is quite worse, poor thing. So I am sending her to Mrs. Gee's for a few days—is it not good of Mrs. G. to have her? She is delightful—she has good qualities, but on too small a scale for this place—and there is a weakness about her which causes me many an evil half hour.

March 22, 1891—Sunday afternoon.

. . . Last night Dr. McDonnell came down to lecture, and Mrs. McD. came in with him. One always feels as if they took a real interest in the hospital and school. Others may feel so, but people are so gauche.

I expect I shall get Agnes some day—perhaps ten years hence. Everything quiet here but as busy as possible. Nurses leave on Thursday, and we are to have no blow out. Committee object to dancing. So the president just gave them their medals and they go.

Miss Quaife's young man has gone off on the bust. So Dr. K. told me this morning. Could she expect anything else? But it is all outside and she is at liberty to make what friends she chooses out of the hospital.

We have three weeks' holiday from class, and I am not sorry. Three nights in the week are tedious.

April 22, 1891.

I received your letters yesterday in which you speak of Gracie's fall. I hope she is all right by this time.

My calls are nearly all paid, but I will make some in my new bonnet. People are nearly always out. Mrs. Girdwood sends me lovely flowers. You say I do not seem happy, and are the committee as good to me? Yes, quite as good. I do not know how it is but really the hospital people spoil me. Still I do not presume on it. I know any day it may change. Of course I am polite to everyone, but they are awfully nice to me. Mrs. Greatorex says I can do anything with any of them, and it is pretty much so. I have got my "comments" just to my mind. Dr. Roddick addresses the nurses!

So you see I am happy—but in the spring hospitals are not nice. One thinks of green places and no people, but one gets over it. I am amused at P. She certainly dreads the "Parrisians". Her idea is a sort of "Asgardian Temple" and I can see she has the elements of wisdom in her plan. But she trembles in her shoes, and my eye, she has got herself up, or rather not got herself up—old grey dress

and old hat, with a dash of crimson in the way of handkerchief. . . .
I went up last night to the cookery school with the nurses—it was
a demonstration—very good. Miss Richards is a good teacher. . . .
Got ideas for Gracie.

Miss Q's young man still goes on the jam. Why she does not
give him G.B. (grand bounce) I do not know. She says: "Miss L.,
what would you do?" I like the "Goddess of Wisdom's" answer
—there is no use in my telling you what I would do; you will not
take my advice, for had I been in your place upon the first offence
I would not forgive him but forget him. She has been very dis-
creet, and after all he was kind to her, and a clever man when
straight. However, as long as she does not throw herself out by a
third storey window! ! ! ! (this last is only in fun of her) I will allow
her to be as miserable as the condition warrants.

Then Mrs. Greatorex's husband has been made a "Knight of
London" one of the rich gifts of the Crown—shelter, food and £100
per annum. When he gets to the top of this tree, or rather when the
top knight dies, the next in order gets 200 per a., living in apartments
in the palace. But it is only for single men. So she pours her little
tub of woe into my sympathetic ear. But she is great fun and we
have lots of laughs over things. Poor thing, she is very plucky—
but you know Q. was so down on Mrs. G. for just what she is doing
herself. I thank goodness that the hen never talks about love
matters.

April 28, 1891.

You have the paper with the "Commencement" exercises.
Everything went off beautifully—the rooms were very nice and
crowded. We went in at a side entrance and at 8 went in two and
two. Miss Q. and Mrs. G. went first, then juniors, seniors, the head
nurses, graduates, and last myself in my black silk and bonnet.
The first four seats were filled with nurses, and they did look lovely—
deep red badges and pincushions. The addresses were short and
sweet. The reporter got everything wrong. . . . It was a nice
dignified ceremony. No singing or nonsense, and as Dr. MacCallum
says, has established a precedent. The tact and finesse I have had
to exercise in the affair so as to please all is a caution. . . .

Our staff go out Friday. Dr. — has had to go to an "inebriate
asylum". Such a nice man, but that one fault. So there is a
vacancy and they say Dr. K. is going to get it. Dr. Roddick likes
him and pushes him forward. We will all miss him—he has been
very good to me—to all of us. I met Mrs. Thomas yesterday and
she was loud in my praise, but she said "Mr. T. was mad they did
not say more about you, for he thinks you are just wonderful, for
it is such a fully equipped and finished school and the Drs. are as
pleased as punch." I said; "Mrs. Thomas, I was glad they said so

little, but I was pleased to hear they appreciated my work." Lily was telling me that little Dr. Birkett was loud in my praises. . . . Sometimes I feel as if I had done nothing. The School cost the hospital the interest of $60,000, but they are all willing and pleased to have it. Dr. K. amuses me. He says it is an established school and will be a success and is, but he is afraid I am going to break down, and then everything will go to pieces. I say *no*. "Bates"(¹) is the only one whose place cannot be filled.

I must tell you for perhaps someone else will, that in December and January we had a regular epidemic of typhoid among the house employees—7 nurses and 7 servants. . . . Thank God everyone got well, but it was an anxious time, for they came down one after the other so quickly. One would get up in the morning and look anxiously for who was missing. As good luck would have it, Nurse Darling, Dr. Craik's protegée and pet, took it, and then Dr. McDonnell and I put in our oar and he, Dr. C., aided and abetted us and the Committee woke up to the drains and they were all seen to, and we had a good overhauling. My eye, what finds ! ! ! —pre-Listerian collections and slops. I can never forget what Dr. McD. was to me and the nurses, and when things were getting better, such eggs and cake and candy and everything good. I always met him smiling and happy. . . . It was at this time that Miss Q. was sent away by Dr. McD. for she had a suspicious tongue, and he said she had better have a change. But it is all over now. Only one nurse went home for any time, and she has not returned. She really was at death's door.

Dr. K. and I had all the responsibility and anxiety. That is when he got provoked at Miss Q. going away, but I had the sense to see it was better so, for she was not afraid, but she had worked hard and was run down. . . . I am very brave about anything infectious —in fact it is no credit to me, for I am not nervous about it. You know of old I never had a nose for bad smells. You see, we were afraid it would injure the school—frighten the probies and so on, but it didn't.

Now I must tell you a tale. You know Dr. McK. is going to be married, and he has always been friendly with everyone, but only *friendly*. Now Nurse Darling, a most efficient nurse, Dr. Craik's pet, thought it would be *very funny* to play a practical joke, and the following will show how it was received by the "Staff".

Saturday evening Dr. McK. asked Miss Q. if she would like to see his present, which consisted of a baby dolly in a crib. Miss Q. was indignant at his even laughing at it and came in and told me— it had been sent down while the staff were at dinner. He *then* knew nothing of who were the senders. But nothing remains a mystery here long, and I found out it was Nurse Darling, and fully knowing

(¹) The steward.

the recent nurses in the house I waited for them to come and confess, which they did.

You may imagine what I said to them. Dr. K. let them know that "The Staff" said it reminded them of the *"bad old times"*. I felt angry enough at the time to have dismissed them, but Dr. K. told me, "Well, if you send Nurse D. away you may make up your mind to go through a Machin experience, for Dr. C. is unscrupulous, and will injure you everywhere"—and it is true, for Dr. McD. and Frank always speak of him as a dangerous man.

So I corrected them and they saw how shocking a thing it was to do. I did not mind Nurse Darling, but their folly hurt me—so sweet a girl. I once heard Nurse Darling speak of me when she did not think I heard her, as "Darling little Nora", so I was beginning to know. Of course Nurse called Mrs. G. queer, but it shows a coarseness which I dislike. . . .

Mrs. T. wants to know if there is any place in Paris where people can be taught dressmaking. She says if anyone undertook an establishment here and did not ask ruinous prices they would coin mun.

May 1, 1891.

M. has just been in to see me. The things are beautiful. My bonnet is most becoming, but the cloak makes me look too immense. I could beat myself that I am not thin. Miss Quaife will jump at it for $15.00. She is so thin. It is such a beauty, oh my, I want it. But I have to confess to too much weight. . . .

We are so upset today. Rooms being cleaned for the Drs. and staff all gone. Dr. Evans looking like a fish out of water. We are giving Dr. K. a lovely clock and doctor's bag with obstetrical instruments. Everyone subscribed in the house, and Dr. Roddick is coming down to present it. Poor Dr. K., he reminds me so much of myself in every way—gets heaps of praise—no brains —all tact and diplomacy—liked and popular—everyone seemingly getting their own way, but in the end doing just as he pleases. We worked well together, and I always felt I could go to him with anything.

I do hate myself sometimes for being so silky to people. Mr. R. came in last night to see me, but Mrs. R., oh, my eye! What a stream what she has done. Some people are so puffed up.

May 4, 1891—Monday.

It has been a very busy day—Monday always is, and the new men are so awkward at first.

The presentation took place Saturday night. Dr. Roddick spoke so nicely—he is always happy in his remarks and so popular with everyone and all classes. The "Staff" men were all speechifying

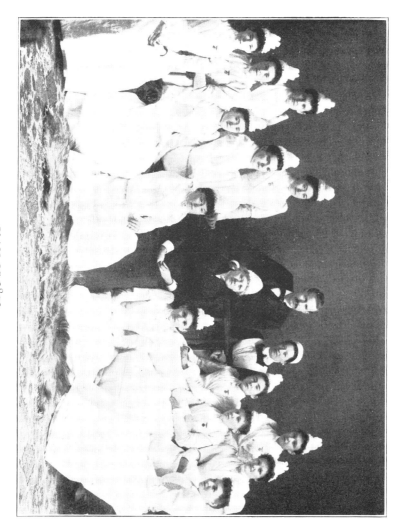

CLASS OF 1893.

Miss Livingston is shown in characteristic pose.

and then Dr. Roddick called on Miss Livingston, but I excused myself. I did have such a hearty laugh over the whole affair—it was so informal—everyone knew each other and Mr. Bates all smiles.

The Committee are thinking of starting a "diet kitchen". We are reorganizing the diet plan used here in prehistoric times. It would be very nice, but unless I can have it as I want it I will not second the move.

Mr. Stirling called on me yesterday with the architect of the "Victoria".(¹) It will not be opened till next May or probably July. No arrangements for surgery, either in the way of operating theatre or beds. I must own I am jealous of that hospital. I would like them to amalgamate, but I fear there is no chance of such a combination, for our pavilions are to be begun soon. . . .

The day the "Sliame" arrived I had a call from an extremely pretty, bright-looking girl, who introduced herself as Miss Warner, Miss C's friend, who had recommended her to me for a position as "charge nurse". I had my doubts. However, I was polite as usual and asked for her testimonials. The next day M. called, and lo, Miss Warner had played rigs on the steamer with Drs. and everybody, besides being an opium eater. So I quashed her in the bud. She said she had a letter to Lady Stanley and has gone to Ottawa. I am becoming like Frank, scary of English nurses who come out here. They are to say the least so selfish, and must be waited on.

Mrs. G. you know thinks of going to Chicago in August. My eye! Will she not have a time spending her money. Just a spirit of adventure makes her think of the move. . . . Mrs. G. is not popular with the Drs. for she is always bothering them with her doubts. But as Dr. K. always said, she was a lady, and the nurses recognize it, never having confidences with the nurses, etc. . . .

Now I want to speak to you about something. I would like to take enough silver—say a couple of forks or one or two teaspoons and have a little communion service—chalice and patin—made for the hospital use. We have none. The one Miss Rimmer had was a disgrace and she took it with her, and I would like to have mamma's and papa's initials put on it. Mr. Evans has a little pocket one. Now, if you do not care to do this why well and good, but I would like to have the service used when I am working. It would be in continual use, for he lives among the dying.

Frank makes me sorry. He is so worried about D. He is a good fellow in the main. So straight in his work and dealings.

May 10, 1891, Sunday.

Nurse Chapman said that the nurses here are all so proud of Miss Livingston—they liked to shew her off. I tell you this for it may

---

(¹) The Royal Victoria Hospital.

please you . . . but do not think I am conceited, for I am not. The nurses should be grateful for I have done much for them and their profession. . . .

I received a nice letter from Lady Stanley today asking if she might adopt our uniform. Certainly the cap and apron I shall send her in miniature, but the pink would not do—she only asks if it would be allowable. Nice note. I really liked Lady Stanley. So unaffected and simple.

What a time! They are tearing down the old buildings. The square is almost open now—it is as good as a play. Such crowds to get the wood and bricks. To see Mr. Bates under all circumstances preserving his good humour is rich. One old woman—"Sir, may I have some wood?" "Yes, madam, I will give you that house in front of you"—and she commences with an axe. The rent from these shacks came to about $12.00 per annum.

Dr. Evans is doing fairly well considering his inexperience—but he is a nice little fellow—neither smokes or drinks. We have now a goody staff. Little Dr. Grafton always says, "Yes, I am well this morning, thank God." But they cannot be too pi for me. Dr. K. was down yesterday afternoon. I was so pleased to see him. I had such a good laugh. It seems Miss Rimmer is very jealous of my success: Frank told me so. She tells Dr. K., "Miss Livingston has maids"—this on account of the pink uniform. He said, "Well, Miss R. you know Miss L. really has been such a success." I have no respect for a woman on her deathbed bearing such malice to a good work. But I always say I feel for Miss R.

You have no idea how Frank is underrated and overlooked, and how Dr. Roddick is always on top of the house. He will be Dean of the Faculty soon or I am much mistaken. The young M.D.'s hang on his word. They respect Frank but find there is no pleasing him. He is good to me. I always have a glass of milk and bread or cake for him when he comes in to operate.

Do not fuss about our having had typhoid. We are all fixed up now. So it did us a good turn. I feel so well and happy. What a strange life to be happy in excitement and change from morning till night. But I have my creature comforts. The food is good and I am well waited on.

Paid a lot of calls yesterday. What common people the R's are. What a vulgar brute. I was charmed with the Blackaders. Such a tasteful and refined looking house and people—but the modern drawing room takes the bun. How you can tell the bringing up. Little Molie (¹) is always killingly polite. His manners are good, at least he knows enough to see you to your cab.

We have had a hot discussion as to allowing lady medical students. Frank at the meeting spoke out like a man. Dr. R. quite

---

(¹) Dr. Molson, on the attending staff.

as much opposed was mum. I have said to both Dr. Craik and Mr. Davidson I do not wish co-education. That mixing of the sexes at lectures is bad and might give rise to complications, when the lady students get strong and brutal. They (the lady students) lost by one vote. I am delighted.

I was so glad to be able to give Frank a nice bowl of soup today. He appreciated it for he did not leave the hospital till 5 p.m.

May 18, 1891—Tuesday.

My dress was sent me on Saturday—rolled in a newspaper and in the pouring rain. The quality of the goods beautiful, but making sloppy—the bill $18.75. I am going to call on Mrs. Gibb as soon as I can get time—they are at the Windsor—one blessing the skirt is light—I am going to pay for it at once. . . .

By the way, Miss Abbott is to be admitted as a student here. There was no way out of it. I am sorry, but being the only one will mind her p's and q's, but we will have to come to it sooner or later.

I was in church on Sunday. Mrs. French([1]) was out when I called, but I met her the other day in the cars—she was very sweet. I think more and more of the R's vulgar house. Why they have not the first pretension to gentility. I am going out there for another afternoon and then I have finished. I like people like the Stirlings and Mr. Routledge. So easy and well bred. Mr. Thomas is always at Lily asking me for a pin and with this closing the flap of her dress, an act which would have sent the R's behind their fans for a week.

May 25, 1891.

. . . Now about my cloak. You must not say it is because no one has one like that that I do not wear or like mine. It is a beauty, but I am fairly choaked up with it and everyone here has one, but this was of silk. Lily would take it but I am deliberating as to a long cloak! through Mrs. Gibb. No! My dress is my *only lesson.* I do not believe they could have given more than $12.00 for it, for the thing is so pitched together—not even made in London, but at Blackheath. One never knows people till they have a money transaction—but I can get it fixed—I have paid them for it but no more of their choosing.

You will be sorry to hear that Dr. McDonnell is far from well—looks awfully—quite broken down—even he owns it. I like him better than any of the Drs.—he is such a gentleman—born not made, and so considerate for everyone. Dr. Evans and I get on very well. Of course I miss Dr. K., but little Evans is a gentleman and

([1]) Wife of the Rev. Arthur French.

can be quite stern with the men servants. Dr. K. has the appointment for the Outdoor. I am so glad he got it instead of Dr. Smith, because Smith is a Bishop's man and disagreeable and a gossip.

Mr. Davidson called on me the day of the meeting—you know he is the "Vic." president. He thinks we are going it too grandly in regard to the "Pavilions". Still, we have the money. He said quite seriously—"Now, Miss Livingston, how would you like to come up to the Victoria, everything spick and span?" You know he is one of the seven trustees. I said, "I cannot give you an answer till I am officially asked." You see, much as I would hate to leave here, for everyone has been so good to me—still, if I could get it I would take the Victoria. Of course the surgery for the next five years will be down here and we will be rich. But the pros and cons are perplexing. I have so many nice probs. that I cannot take them all.

Miss Q. with all her weakness for Mr. "jim jams" is so valuable. She never asks for off time. The hospital comes first even in her pleasures—it is so funny to live with two such dissimilar characters as she and Mrs. G.

June 7, 1891, Sunday.

. . . It is the same routine day after day, and the time flies by so quickly. Before one payroll is made up the next is preparing. We have been very busy—nurses taking holidays, but we have a good full staff this year. Mrs. G. takes her vacation the first week in July. She thinks now she will go only down the Saguenay. Miss Q. will no doubt go to New York and home by the St. Lawrence.

I got your letter yesterday and was amused at the "kind"—our friend Q. gives vent to such explosions. I did not even see that M.B. took any prize at the art exhibition—her name was not even mentioned. Why, I could not imagine myself refined about the B's. They were fairly dragged up.

I tell you what I would like—a blue tailor-made dress—and a blue bonnet, made like my grey and lined in the same way, with flower to complete. I should like it for this fall.

Mrs. Greatorex is in great trouble. Her husband tells her if he can get a divorce he can marry a girl, niece of the M's of Breadalbane, with £4,000 per year—oh, he is a scamp, and she would be well rid of him.

. . . My nurses are all busy. They are nursing two and two—day and night—pretty good for Montreal.

June 12, 1891.

. . . I got a note from Dr. McDonnell—he is in a bad way. Frank ordered him off at once. I am losing my best friend. Of course Frank is kindness itself. . . . Then poor Dr. Kirkpatrick. Took suddenly ill—was down here Saturday morning—went home and took a bad hæmorrhage. The hospital has killed him—though after he left he picked up wonderfully. Frank and Dr. Roddick say his only chance is in not having a consumptive family history. . . . I am very sorry—I will miss him. Dr. E. and I get on very well yet he cannot compare to Dr. K. Of course his management does not affect me—only reflects on himself—such as rudeness—well, not exactly that, but shortness to applying patients. Now Dr. K. was something like myself—would sympathize almost to tears— but he held his own and bowed them out pleased with *themselves.* It is a training this institution life. Two ladies full of good works and human failings called on me the other day just as Mrs. G. and I were going out. She was put out and shewed it. I had all the talking to do and convincing—and after they left Mrs. G. said, "Why, Miss L. how you smoothed them down. I really thought they must be friends—you seemed so considerate of their feelings."

My last year's satin has been ironed and looks so nicely. My black bonnet—the old one—is so much admired. Frank always calls it "The Lady Stanley".

June 19, 1891.

. . . You know Nurse Hall has left and I am delighted. Dr. T., Bishop's College, asked her to step a little more briskly— he is one of the new staff and as bumptious as Hall herself. So she sent in her resignation which I accepted. Then her old father was in a wax and now would like to get her into the "Maternity" for six months. They are most disagreeable, disputatious, step-on-your-toes people. Dr. McDonnell told me all about the family. I am glad that I am rid of her. What character one strikes in a community of 40 women.

. . . I went up to see Dr. K. He looks very badly. Still I am not so blue in my diagnosis as Dr. and Mrs. McDonnell. Poor fellow, he made me quite sad. We will miss him in the Outdoor, but I am glad to have Drs. McKechnie and Brown in his place and not a Bishop's man—I do not like them. Dr. K. goes to the mountains. I am glad he did not take ill when he was here, for he is so comfortable where he is.

Frank had such a nice man with him Friday, Dr. Stilwell, St. Malo, California. He has a small hospital—25 patients—and wants a superintendent and matron combined—gives $50 per month. I introduced him to Nurse Donnovan and I think in all probability she will go out with him in May next. He will allow her to have her little boy with her, which is an object! She is extremely pretty and nice mannered. He was very much pleased with her. She is a fine ward runner and thoroughly trustworthy. There is no doubt about a nurse getting paying work if she is equal to it.

June 26, 1891.

. . . Dr. K. has had more hæmorrhages. Mrs. G. was up there this morning. Really, English people are *awful*. She wanted him to give her a "testimonial" and of course if she had any tact she would see that her going for it looks as if she was afraid he might slip off. But they are so selfish—they only look at everything as it betters or injures themselves.

July 23, 1891.

. . . Como did look lovely, but I am always glad to get home again. Our dinner was waiting for us and the most lovely flowers— one enormous bunch of sweet peas, sent me by Florrie Shaw, L's cousin at Perth. . . . Do not think I am becoming giddy when I tell you that Dr. Evans took Mrs. G. and I for a drive the other evening. It was so unselfish of him, for the pleasure was all on our side. I could not have refused going. We drove round the two mountains, and the sweet smells and green lawns were so refreshing. I get on very well with him—his mistakes are in admonishing patients without judgment—without asking me in many cases, when I could help him. He has, and I have let him, come down with some pretty hard bumps. But he is a nice gentlemanly boy— in fact, they are all nice—but not *very* clever—not like the old staff.

July 30, 1891.

. . . Poor Dr. McD. is very low. Frank is there day and night —he is just tired out. Lily came down on Monday to see Dr. Brown. I hope he will do her some good. I do not think he is a very clever man not to have seen her condition long ago. My opinion of Montreal *medical* men is not very high.

Dr. and Mrs. Carmichael called on me yesterday, but I was out. I can tell you if you go to church twice anywhere but at St. John's they call on you at once. The sisters have taken to coming to see me vigorously, but it is rather late in the day.

A very great opera is running here and has been for the last two months. 75c. is not dear for the best seats, do you think so? I am going tonight with Mrs. Greatorex, for the first time. She is a very nice companion—the Brocks were charmed with her, and since I have got to know her she improves. It is such a comfort to have a lady to talk to, and she is full of fun too.

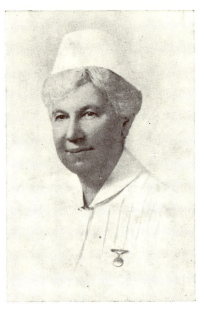

MISS JANE WEBSTER
Night Superintendent from 1900-1933.

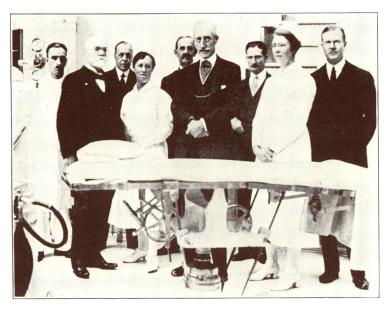

A GROUP IN THE OPERATING ROOM ON ONE OF
LORD WILLINGDON'S VISITS.

From left to right: Dr. C. C. Stewart; Dr. F. J. Shepherd; Dr. A. T. Bazin; Miss I. Davies; Dr. F. G. Finley; Lord Willingdon; an aide; Miss F. Strumm; Colonel Herbert Molson.

August 11, 1891.

. . . Just came in from Miss Rimmer's funeral. Poor Frank, he is having a mournful time of it lately. I expect he will have Agnes by and by. . . . Yes, I think it would be nice if I could be with you, but you must think of me here as happy as happy can be. There is no doubt my vocation is a hospital. It is a pity everyone does not find the place they were made for.

. . . I wish you could see our pavilions—gorgeous. I gaze at them lovingly, for I am proud of them. If I did go to the "Victoria" it would be a wrench. I think the Committee are a little uneasy as to the R.V.

We have a project on foot, Mr. Thomas and I for getting the nurses an outdoor blue cloak and bonnet, the cloak having a cross something like an ambulance cross. All are delighted to hear it— they really will look so charming in it that I said to Dr. Spier, "someone will have to go about with them." He said "I will undertake the position." The Staff are all such nice boys—flirt less even than the last did.

August 12, 1891.

. . . Had a dreadful fright yesterday. I was sitting in my room when I heard someone running towards my room. Dr. E. opened the door as I did, and said "Miss Livingston, the hospital is on fire! !" For a moment I felt as if I should collapse. I asked where, and if he had rung for the reels—in two seconds I was in "33"— you could see the fire through the ventilator from the chimney. By this time, the whole street in front was packed with engines, salvage waggons, etc.

It was soon put out but the firemen stayed for three or four hours. The worst of it was the engineers and Bates were both out on business. An overheated chimney. The day was one like the day in Como, when we had the coal fricas! ! Had Nurse Prime not had presence of mind—getting up quietly when she saw the fire, and not disturbing the patients, we might have had a panic. Luckily, she met Dr. E. in the hall. I might just as well have been in alone as not, for I often am—I mean, Dr. E. etc. have to go out. Poor Bates was in Mr. Davidson's office when he heard the telephone ring the fire alarm for the Hospital—he was in a stew.

But all is well that ends well, and now all the chimneys are to be cleaned. There is no doubt the loss of life in case of fire would be large, even though method and coolness were observed. Dr. E. is as fussy as I am. He had the watchman on the roof in the night in case of anything.

I had a lovely letter from Mrs. McDonnell. I am glad I was a comfort—that good soul now gone . . . .

The Committee are considering the wearing of an outdoors uniform for the nurses. They presented such a motley appearance at Dr. McD's funeral—the Committee want to be proud of them—dark blue shirred cloak and bonnet. I told you something of this before, but it is I think pretty sure. The nurses are delighted. How proud I will be of them. Dr. E. says "dangerously nice", and that I will need a watchdog, an M.D. preferred, to look after them.

. . . They say Lily McD. is trying for the "Victoria" but they will have to wait for her till Fall. One hears so many reports of all kinds. Frank always says if I should leave here I would never get such a nice position, meaning I do as I will, and no one interferes with me. Poor F. I am sorry for him. He is so bothered by L's illness and he is a good friend, but not one scrap of influence.

August 20, 1891.

Agnes sent me word she would see me at Dr. S. So I went up and she is to come to me . . . Mrs. Molson wanted her to go to "Verdun Asylum" but Agnes preferred coming to the M.G.H. She is so nice. She is taking lessons at the "Cookery School" . . . She will be a great comfort to me.

. . . When Q. was away I was up at 6 a.m. and busy I can tell you. But everyone is good and kind to me and very considerate. Nurse Alicia helped me in so many ways. By the way, I would like a pretty something for her—not expensive, say a pretty photo. You know she gave me a pretty handkerchief case at Xmas. Mrs. Greatorex goes to Chicago in October. Nurse Baikie is to take her position—much better than she is. But a night nurse at $8.00 instead of $35.00 would make a precedent, and I might not always have so capable a nurse as Nurse B. She did beautifully when Mrs. G. was away—gas bill $20.00 less during the month.

Mrs. Grindlay came to see me with Nurse Carvell, who is taking care of her. Nice woman, but almost crazy with nerves. Nurse had a soft snap of it. The graduates mind me and do just as I say, much more than the majority of nurses did in New York. I could place four for every one out now—everyone has a trained nurse now for everything and nothing.

August 27, 1891, Thursday.

Mrs. Greatorex leaves Oct. 1st for Chicago. She is a pleasant companion, but as a nurse nil. She has such a nervous manner that when the Drs. are sick they beg not to have her take them medicine or poultices. Nurse Baikie will take her position for a time—so competent and dignified. But if I once allow the Committee to pay only $8.00 instead of $35.00 per month they will think my class must provide a night supt.

P. has not been in this week as she intended. Mind you, I do not for a moment think Miss H. and she will pull—and if she falls out, what will happen, for no one will come on for what she can give—it is a big risk for her—I would like you to have classes there if possible, but not to be sat on, as only a fool like she can sit. I hate a puffed-up person—blatant ass. I wish you could hear Mrs. Greatorex describe M. Popham's ideas of Miss P. painting! ! !

Had visit from Dr. K. who is on at the hospital again. Dr. Birkett was telling me the other day Dr. K's case was just Dr. McD. over again.

I have had a tiring week—everything wrong. I had to send a nurse away, just for cussedness—it is lovely now she has gone, and I was determined she should go. Then I had to speak to one of the doctors for flirting with a nurse. They certainly give me little trouble that way and are so nice when I do speak. I have no lack of moral courage. I wish everyone could be as dignified as I am, but people are so foolish and lose their balance so easily.

Sept. 7, 1891.

I hear that Dr. Craik is ill. Really, what ails the M.D.'s? Poor Dr. McD.—how I miss him. . . .

I think you are coming out a little late. However, it makes no difference . . . I suppose you have the only K. in Canada. That babe in arms, Phillips—to think with my experience she could beguile me into sending up the K. to Shepherd's rooms! ! ! let alone her tricks—the risk from fire and seizure. No, No, P., your little plot kicked the beam. I daresay she would have supervised the putting up and then cooked her lunch in it! ! ! . . . How many things I will have to tell you that take too long to write. I will be glad to get a rest. I feel well, but I want to get away from people—doctors and nurses—but only for a time.

May 13, 1897.

. . . I must tell you that Nurse Alicia has kicked for higher salary, and the Committee accepted her resignation—so good. Miss Tedford is engaged, for which I am well pleased.

In addition to these extracts it has been thought worth while to give examples of her remarks on some of the nurses who passed through her hands in the School. Up to 1899 Miss Livingston kept a record of all the nurses and made comments on each one of them. These of course, were for her own private institution records, and must remain so. But there can be no harm in quoting a few of them to give an idea of her insight into character.

Miss Baikie—Able, level head. *Very confident.* Pretty.

. . . .—Very Imprudent.

. . . .—Satisfactory—fussy—*most reliable.*

. . . .—Forth-putting—fond of gossip. Unprofessional.

. . . .—No force, no endurance. Pleasing personally.

. . . .—Professionally good nurse. Socially untrue. Loud—fond of admiration.

. . . .—Most reliable—no polish. Good staying power.

. . . .—Faithful, discrete, loyal. Popular with all.

. . . .—Careful, slow, stubborn. Needs a master.

. . . .—Slow—always aggrieved.

. . . .—Tactless—old maidish *very.*

. . . .—Hands—no head.

. . . .—Fairly good nurse—needs handling—inclined to flirt, etc.

. . . .—Superior education — nervous — a lady in every thought.

. . . .—Good nurse. A little too sympathetic. Superior education. Exceptional in theory. To be trusted.

. . . .—Faults those of previous environment. Very aggressive. Manner will improve in private practice and with training.

. . . .—Very Irish! ! ! Good and true. *Good sleeper.*

. . . .—Selfish. Reliable. No enthusiasm—in fact, a *commercial nurse.*

. . . .—Very good operating room nurse. "Very attentive to the staff." Principles nil.

. . . .—Faults those of environment. Disagreeable voice for sick room.

. . . .—Accurate. *Dense.*

. . . .—Asked to resign. *Gossip.*

............—Fond of admiration and notice. Very neurotic but principles fine.

............—Does not wear well.

............—Excellent faithful nurse.

............—Disobeyed and broke rules regarding doctors, etc. Confessed.

............—Superior education. Manner apathetic—no jump. *True. Discrete* as to things seen and heard.

............—Principles not perfect.

............—Set upon herself, but accurate.

APPENDIX B

THE ALUMNAE ASSOCIATION OF
THE MONTREAL GENERAL HOSPITAL

A most important outgrowth of the School has been the Alumnae Association. The need for such an organization was recognized for some time and in 1905, at the instance of Miss M. L. Parker, Miss Livingston called a general meeting of graduates to discuss the matter. The meeting was held on April 17, in the Governors' Hall, and a large number of nurses assembled. Some of those present were the Misses Dodds, Jennie Webster, S. E. Young, Flora Strumm, M. L. Parker, May Young, M. F. Mc-Cutcheon and Nora Tedford.

Miss Livingston announced that Miss Parker would explain the object of the meeting. Miss Parker stated that her idea was to form a club for the benefit of the graduate nurses, the need being quite evident. She felt too that later on an alumnae organization might be built up. The plan was well received and an organization was duly formed. The original suggestion to call it the "Livingston Club" was vetoed by Miss Livingston herself, and it was then called "The M.G.H. Graduate Nurses Club". The club house (probably the first of its kind in Canada) was on Park Avenue, and served its purpose well for some years.

In 1909, however, Miss F. M. Shaw pointed out that the organization was to all intents and purposes an alumnae association, and the name was accordingly changed to "The Alumnae Association of the M.G.H. Training School". The constitution states the object to be "The promotion of unity and good fellowship among its members, the advancement of the profession of nursing, and of making provision for its nurses when ill or disabled."

One of the most valuable activities of the Association has been the formation of a Sick Benefit Fund for nurses. This came into being almost entirely through the vision and efforts of Miss Nora Tedford. Various methods were used for collecting money for it, such as a "Weighing Party", and a bazaar, which were supplemented by gifts from friends, including many of the doctors. The help and advice of Dr. E. M. Eberts were of great value in investment and by 1917 the Fund became available. It renders financial assistance

114

to sick members by supplying private ward accommodation in the hospital and assuming responsibility for any special fee incurred.

The Association also carries on a regular educational programme of addresses for its members each year.

The fiftieth anniversary of the founding of the Training School was celebrated at a special meeting of the Alumnae Society, held in the Nurses' Home on the evening of Thursday, February 22nd, 1940. This was as close to the actual day of the month on which Miss Livingston arrived at the hospital as could be arranged. Some curtailment of the celebrations had been necessary on account of the war, but nevertheless the proceedings were lively and impressive. The large numbers of graduates in attendance far exceeded expectations, and the hall was filled to overflowing.

The president of the Association, Miss Mary Mathewson, was in the chair, and she had on the platform with her Miss Mabel Holt, lady superintendent, Miss Flora Strumm, assistant superintendent, and Miss Agnes Tennant, secretary of the Association. A notable guest of honour was also there in the person of Miss Jennie Webster, former night superintendent.

A very interesting historical contrast had been arranged by dressing one of the undergraduate nurses (Miss Margaret Browne) in a uniform of the same material first used in the School, a pink and white (and by now much faded) striped material, very fragile in its old age. Every detail of the uniform was complete, down to the chatelaine worn at the waist. Beside her sat another undergraduate (Miss Eileen Sherlock) dressed in the modern uniform.

After a slight sensation caused by Miss Webster falling off the platform backwards, as she moved her chair, the meeting was opened by Miss Mathewson, with some excellent explanatory and welcoming remarks. It was regretted that the one living member of the first graduating class, Miss Christina Mackay, of Martintown, Ont., could not be present. She had been called on a case at the last moment. It was an evidence of her vigour which received admiring comment.

Miss Strumm received an ovation which unmistakably indicated her personal popularity with the many graduates who have been taught under her. In spite of much persuasion to make a speech she could not be induced to do more than accept a place on the platform.

The programme consisted in the main of a series of short speeches by various graduates and members of the hospital staff. These were in the nature of reminiscences of the early days of the School, and of Miss Livingston and others associated with her.

Some of the speakers took considerable pains in committing their remarks to writing, notably Miss Annie Colquhoun and Miss Henrietta Dunlop.

Miss Colquhoun spoke with a vivacity and humour which are not to be readily reproduced.

MISS COLQUHOUN'S ADDRESS

May I say how happy I am to be with you tonight after more than 25 years in California, meeting my old friends among the doctors and nurses, and through the Alumnae those of the younger generation.

I have so much to say: so I thought it better to write it down lest I become garrulous. I see Miss Johns of the *Canadian Nurse* is here. She says if we have anything to write "Boil it down and keep on boiling". I have endeavoured to do so, and you may find it a bit thick in spots and much left out.

I see also Miss Jean Wilson, our secretary of the Canadian Nurses' Association, which is a federation of our nine provinces and represents 15,600 registered nurses in the Dominion. When I called upon her in her office last year I did not know that I had ever met her until she said "I saw you when I was six years of age in your lovely pink uniform and then and there decided I was going to be a nurse, went home, put all my dolls to bed, and here I am due to your unconscious influence." I find life full of surprises.

I feel that this grand old M.G.H. is like the hub of a wheel, the spokes radiating to all corners of the earth.

I entered the hospital in April 1890, came up from the Grand Trunk station in a cab, passing the horse-drawn street cars with their tinkling bells. I arrived with mingled feelings, was received graciously by Miss Livingston and assigned to the children's ward, where Miss Christie Mackay reigned supreme. She was an excellent nurse and instructress, and told me if I were never seen sitting down I would be more sure of getting my cap. Faith! I never had time to sit down, as there were always dressings to make and bandages to roll, white for Dr. Shepherd and pink for Dr. Bell.

After four months in the children's ward I was sent to Ward 11, the men's medical, situated where the Governor's Hall is now. I went on day duty until I learned the ropes, then was put on night duty, scared to death with the responsibility. No orderly, only little me, with as many as eight to ten typhoids to be sponged q.2.h. if temperatures were over 102 2/5; pneumonia patients with double jacket, linseed poultices q.4.h. Mrs. Greatorex, the night superintendent, came q.3.h.

I got through somehow, thanks to the Lord and convalescent patients were kind and helped with A.M. ablutions. Miss Livingston's "Nurse, I am pleased with your work while on night duty" when I had finished was compensation enough for me.

My greatest terror at night was the rats! Miss Macgregor, my classmate, said to me before writing this, "You are not going to speak about the rats! I saw but one." "Yes," I replied, "there was a man who lived all his life in India and never saw a tiger". RATS!! A stamp of the foot when turning up the gas in the kitchens sent them and the cockroaches scurrying. One of my duties was to telephone Dr. R. E. McKechnie when one got in a trap, as he wanted them for research work. They ate our gloves, shoes and handkerchiefs. One day on going to my room I saw a tail gracefully hanging out of a bureau drawer. That was just too much. I seized a pair of curling tongs, clamped them over said tail and shouted for assistance. Nurses arrived with brooms and boots, and believe it or not, we killed *that* rat. I venture to think that they and the bedbugs may have been responsible for the many cases of erysipelas in our surgical wards after operation.

The Misses Cooper and Cashen were my room-mates in the north-east corner, all still alive. Across the hall were my good friends Alma Bush and Miss Baikie, who always did good work wherever she was placed, and Charlotte Hetherington, all gone now. Charlotte eloped with Dr. Wade from the Maternity Hospital. Thereafter we were not even allowed to *speak* to a student. The papers made much of it and said, "Lovely M.G.H. nurse elopes with medical student. Mothers fear to send their sons to McGill lest they be trapped by wily nurses."

Miss Johns, I have boiled and boiled and now will have to let the residue settle and skim off a few facts. I did want to speak of typhoid and tell you of the emergency hospital on Aqueduct Street and the good work done there, but the clock says no. I see Dr. Patch who was in charge there and he can tell you about it.

Last Saturday's *Star* had a cut of the operating room, with three of the doctors and Miss Collins. I can visualize it in 1890 with its rows of students on the benches, and up in the corner Dr. Maude Abbott and Dr. Ritchie England, our first lady medical students. Nurse Alicia Dunne in charge was a bit of a martinet, a stickler for surgical cleanliness, and nothing missed her eagle eye. I am glad to have trained under her.

I want to speak, in passing, of the last time I saw Dr. Tait McKenzie in Edinburgh, when he came over for the tenth anniversary of the placing of his statue of the Scottish American soldier. Many of you have seen it—"The Call"—the eager Highland lad with his rifle across his knees, facing Edinburgh Castle, will always be a memorial to Scotland's sons as well as to Canada's sons, and we may well be proud of him and of all our grand doctors who have distinguished themselves. Dr. Tait came in with the Countess of Aberdeen on his arm (he had served as their medical officer while in Ottawa). I had a word with each of them, and now they too have joined the great majority. I wish you could have heard the pipes and seen the Duke of Athol in his kilt.

Then another spoke from our hub was meeting Dr. Ritchie of the M.G.H. x-ray department, whom I had never met, but learned they lived next door to my fellow graduate, Mrs. Pearson, in Montreal West.

I spent two years with my friend Miss Cooper, in her Devon home near Torquay, set in a lovely old garden with primroses under the hedge. We had long evenings reading aloud before the open fire. One day Miss Emma Cooper brought home from the library a Life of Dr. Shepherd (by Dr. W. B. Howell, who used to be anæsthetist at the M.G.H.). How we did enjoy it—another M.G.H. link.

But I must hasten on. The two years sped quickly by, and we were ready for graduation. Miss Livingston's parting words to our class will never be forgotten: "Young ladies, you are the pioneers in the field of professional nursing. It will be your task to educate the public and to blaze the trail for those who will follow you. Many of the untrained nurses have been eating with the maids. Make arrangements, when you enter a home, to have your meals served on a tray. Be dignified and wise, and remember you have your Training School and the M.G.H. at your back." Wise counsel. And we did blaze the trail, and though we may not have cut a wide swath or road, we followed the straight and narrow path.

I think, like Solomon, a nurse should ask the Lord for an understanding heart, as well as a sense of humour. We who welcome the new life and close the eyes of those who enter the "Great Adventure" need kind hearts. Of all the ministries of our Lord I like best to read John's act—in Moffatt's version—when the disciples had toiled all night and caught nothing, at break of day saw on the shore a charcoal fire with fish cooking thereon and bread. And the Master said, "bring more fish and come and breakfast". How very human it was, and we through Him who "was kind to the unthankful and to the evil" minister today. And He is not far from those who "while others sleep, are toiling upward in the night".

By our training in this hospital we have been marked to do something worth-while in this world. And I say God bless the Montreal General Hospital and all the nurses and doctors who have served in it before and after the past fifty years. Great things are expected of us, for we have been given much.

117

The next speaker was Miss Jennie Webster, who was received with the greatest enthusiasm. She spoke with all her old vigour and emphasis, and recalled many events in her nursing career which caused much amusement and interest. These began with a description of her first day in the ward, when she was repeatedly and solemnly warned to do nothing that she had not been told to do. These instructions she carried out to the letter. So much so, that in getting a patient ready for a teaching clinic, she sent him off in the bed, without a nightshirt, because, as she calmly informed the infuriated head nurse later on, "she hadn't been told to put one on."

Miss Webster recalled that the outdoor department was always a lively place, especially on Saturday nights. The streets around the hospital, especially Cadieux and St. Dominique, were apt to be very tumultuous at times. Sometimes, if the brawling became intolerable she would go out on the verandah and call out to them, and sometimes even went down to tell them they must stop. She was well known to all of them, for there were few who hadn't been through the outdoor department at some time or other. And she never had any trouble in quelling their rioting.

Her night work was always hard, but always interesting. When she took over there was only one night orderly, a Swede called Janie, and he did everything for everybody. Miss Webster remembers giving as many as 33 typhoid baths in a night. "In the morning," she said, "my arms were as long as my legs, and I was so tired that I wouldn't have run from a bear." Typhoid, of course, used to fill the wards to overflowing. Miss Strumm was one of the nurses who contracted the disease, and Miss Webster recalled that her temperature went as high as 107.

Miss Webster spoke with a full heart about Miss Livingston's extraordinary personality. It was she who brought out the best in her nurses, because she gave herself so freely.

Miss Henrietta Dunlop then followed, with the following address.

MISS DUNLOP'S ADDRESS

On December 11, 1890, I went to see the formal opening of the Montreal General Hospital Training School for Nurses by the Governor-General, Lord Stanley and Lady Stanley, at the Windsor Hotel.

When I saw how nice the nurses all looked in their pink uniforms and starched aprons, I thought it would be a fine thing to be one of them. Everyone discouraged my going into the M.G.H. Dr. Edward Williams and Dr. John Hewittson both said how dirty the place was and overrun by rats and that it was no place for a young girl. I think they graduated about the time Miss Livingston came. Other people told me what horrid things I would have to do; one was that I would have to wash a dead nigger! Fancy all the niggers waiting to die to accommodate probationers! However, after seeing Miss Livingston whose personality and direct way of speaking reassured me, I entered my nursing career in April 1891 at the age of eighteen years. When one thinks of what Miss Livingston

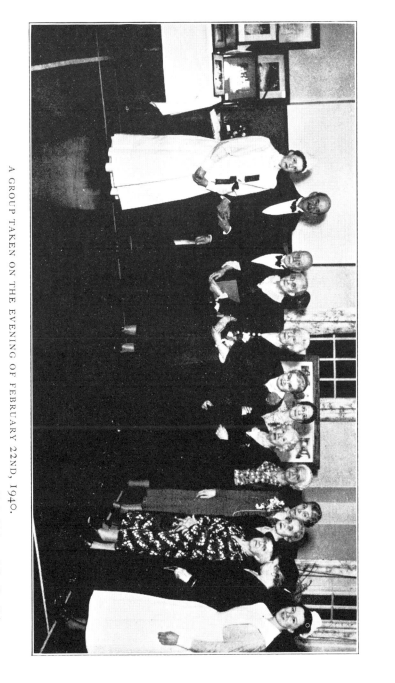

A GROUP TAKEN ON THE EVENING OF FEBRUARY 22ND, 1940.

From left to right: Miss M. Browne in the original uniform of the school; Dr. F. G. Finley; Dr. H. S. Birkett; Miss DesBrisay; Miss Webster; Dr. Maude E. Abbott, one of the first women students at the hospital; Mrs. Pearson; Miss A. Colquhoun; Mrs. Dunfield; Miss Dunlop; Miss Sullivan; Miss Colley; Mrs. Henderson; Miss Eileen Sherlock, in the modern uniform.

accomplished in one year it is hard for any one now to realize what that meant, but the first and second classes saw it, as they were right inside while the changes were being made. Wet sheets hanging over the banisters, cuspidors in the men's wards, night nurses sleeping on duty and patients with fractured legs getting out of bed to reach their stimulants on the shelf above them. One thing we never liked was carrying the bed spring out to the bathroom and putting each end into boiling water in the bath. When a patient had been in for some time we had sufficient evidence that he or she had had many visitors at night. Having no orderlies to fetch and carry for us, *that* had to be done by the nurses besides many other things nurses nowadays do not have to do.

The bathrooms were awful, especially the one in Ward Eleven and we had to clean them besides polishing the brass taps, the tin tubs and dust the wards and corridors.

Miss Livingston brought with her two graduates from the New York Hospital, Miss Quaife as Assistant to Miss Livingston and Miss Collyer as Night Supervisor. Miss Collyer only stayed six months and was followed by Mrs. Greatorex, a graduate, I think, of St. Thomas's Hospital of London, England. She was a very severe disciplinarian. Miss Baikie succeeded her in two years. Miss Quaife was succeeded by Miss Davis, an English graduate. Unlike us, she wore very short, starched skirts, bound round with navy blue braid and cap with ties under the chin, large white apron and bib. Nurse Alicia Dunn, though she trained for a year under Miss Livingston, did not wear the pink uniform. She had charge of the operating room and wore a black dress with white apron, a small bib and no cap. We were just told by Miss Quaife in the morning to report in the O.R. by ten or eleven o'clock. If we had time we would run up to our room on the top floor, which was the nurses' quarters, and change our apron and go to the operating room in the same uniform we had worn in the wards for days. Nurse Mary Collins was the one who was more often sent. She preferred it to the wards. After the surgical wings were built, Nurse Alicia left and Miss Tedford took charge and very ably ran it until after the Great War.

Miss Livingston held all our classes and we had lectures from the doctors about every second week in the evenings. In 1906, Miss F. M. Shaw, Class 1896, was appointed as the first Instructress of the Training School, another of Miss Livingston's achievements. We had cooking classes, too, once a week, before the Diet Kitchen was established. That was in 1896 and in 1897 Miss Gracie Livingston was appointed dietitian, in which office she continued until her retirement in 1920.

We had an outdoor uniform, a navy blue cloak covering all our pink uniform and a small bonnet with a blue Alsatian bow and blue and white ribbons tied under the chin. As this uniform was not compulsory it was soon given up when new nurses took our places.

Viola Hersey, now Mrs. Henderson, was my head assistant and Miss Jennie Webster my probationer. The former served during the last war and for many succeeding years as Lady Superintendent of the St. John's Ambulance Brigade; the latter, as you all know, was night superintendent of the M.G.H. for over thirty years.

The obstetrical course was not compulsory. The old Maternity Hospital was on St. Urbain Street below Dorchester, another very old building, and Miss Emily Cooper was in charge of it, after she graduated in 1892.

It was only a two year course then and there were many wards to go through besides the Outdoor Department. Time does not allow me to tell of that Outdoor Department in the basement but there are many here who will remember it and good work was done there under many drawbacks.

When I graduated and was entitled to the fee of two dollars per day on private duty, considered a large sum in those days, I went first of all into the Contagious Wards; on the diphtheria floor Dr. Hubert Hamilton was the visiting doctor with Dr. John Spier as his assistant. Children would be brought in with their throats closed and choking. Intubation had to be performed at once to save their lives, but in many cases not successfully. The Infectious Wards were in an

119

old building on Cadieux Street side. Miss Livingston came for my report each day. She talked to me through a small shutter in a door connecting with the main building. She was my only contact with the outside world besides the doctors.

Before closing I would like to say that I am glad to have Miss Sullivan here tonight as she is the only representative of our class besides myself. Mrs. Carmichael, nee Jessie Bolster, regrets not being with us and sends greetings to any doctors and nurses who may remember her. Thinking of these old days so long ago, I think I hear Miss Livingston say "Nurse—the PATIENT—always the patient first." I think that spirit still lives within these old walls.

Mrs. John Henderson (Viola Hersey, 1894), Mrs. Dunfield (Miss Lepoidevin) and Miss Georgina Colley (1895) all added their reminiscences. Miss Colley (on whom Miss Livingston's comment in her class book was "Superior woman and nurse") referred to her experiences with the doctors on the staff with a naiveté which threw the audience into convulsions of laughter.

Several of the medical staff were present who had been in the hospital at the time and even before the Training School was started. Dr. H. S. Birkett, who was the oldest remaining member of the staff, spoke briefly about his memories of the nurses of the early days. Some of them, he said, were typical "Sairey Gamps", and to the great delight of the audience he described an encounter he had with one of them in the ward, when he was a student.

He was sitting on the side of a bed talking to a patient, when he heard a curt order from the nurse at the head of the ward to "get off that bed". He paid no attention to what he could not believe was meant for him, and soon the command was repeated, this time with the added threat "or I'll throw you off". "Come and try," said Dr. Birkett, and in a moment a wrestling match was in full progress. The patients entered into the spirit of the thing and odds were freely offered on the doctor. However, superior weight eventually told and the nurse was victorious. To show that there was no ill-feeling some years later she called in Dr. Birkett to see her, and he found her to be in the last stages of tuberculosis. But she still recalled their previous encounter with relish.

Dr. F. G. Finley then paid his tribute to Miss Livingston's powers of administration, and also spoke of some of the men who had helped to raise and maintain the high standards of the hospital. Dr. W. F. Hamilton followed. He pointed out that the development of the institution measured in influence with the ramifications of business, social and spiritual life. Dr. C. F. Martin spoke of the atmosphere of the hospital as being rich in memories. He had always been impressed with the fact that Miss Livingston sought especially to develop initiative in her nurses.

Dr. A. T. Bazin confined himself chiefly to recalling two outstanding figures in the nursing life of the hospital, Miss Alicia Dunne and Miss Jennie Webster. His reminiscences of Miss Dunne have already been referred to (page 50). He spoke of his work in the infectious diseases hospital, with Miss Webster, who was in charge of it, and paid tribute to her sterling qualities of dependability and shrewdness. He recalled that one short year after its opening, the nursing school was functioning as smoothly and efficiently as if it had always been there. This was entirely due to the guidance of Miss Livingston.

Special mention was also made of Miss Nora Tedford, who had succeeded Miss Dunne in charge of the operating room, and had a splendid record of efficient and self-effacing work for 21 years. Miss Tedford was in the audience, but could not be induced to speak of her work.

The whole evening was one of warm-hearted tribute to Miss Livingston's creation of the nursing school out of what could only be called chaos. She needed energy, courage, tact and strength of character. All these she possessed, and to them she added a kindliness which was all the more appreciated because it was never paraded, as well as an unfailing sense of humour which must have often been needed. But she was always thinking of her nurses, and was always ready to fight for their rights. Her justice and fairness of dealing were never questioned. Naturally, she attracted the best possible type of woman to her school, and the outstanding qualities of those whom she had on her staff are all well recognized.

This commemoration laid before the present generation the story of a fine achievement. Miss Livingston was the central figure, but those who supported her and followed her example received their due meed of honour.

An additional feature of the evening was a historical display which was open to view after the meeting. Photographs of the old wards and of the hospital were shown, together with some old instruments and apparatus of great interest. Prominent among these was the carbolic spray which Dr. Roddick brought to the hospital as part of the antiseptic ritual first practised. The charter of the hospital was on display, with some of the original minute books and other records of the hospital.

APPENDIX C

GRADUATES OF THE MONTREAL GENERAL HOSPITAL SCHOOL OF NURSING AND THE WESTERN HOSPITAL SCHOOL FOR NURSES

The Alumnae Associations of these two Schools amalgamated
by mutual consent and agreement, in October, 1933

MONTREAL GENERAL HOSPITAL

Class 1891

Carroll, Georgina (deceased)
Chapman, Ellen A. (deceased)
Dunn, Alicia (deceased)
English, Julia (deceased)
MacKay, Christina (deceased)
Preston, Jessie (Mrs. P. H. Gregory) (deceased)

Class 1892

Annand, Mary (Mrs. A. Robertson) (deceased)
Baikie, Elizabeth (deceased)
Burton, Eugenie (deceased)
Bush, Alma E. (Mrs. A. E. Rolph) (deceased)
Cashen, Alice (Mrs. A. Gilmore) (deceased)
Collins, Mary (married) (deceased)
Colquhoun, Annie (deceased)
Connor, Bessie (Mrs. S. Barker) (deceased)
Cooper, Emily (deceased)
Darling, Effie (deceased)
Haggart, Barbara (deceased)
Hobday, Ethel M. (married) (deceased)
Howes, Harriet (married) (deceased)
Jackson, Margaret (Mrs. M. Archer)
Jolly, Nora (Mrs. L. Girdwood)
MacGregor, Jessie (deceased)
Merser, Emma (deceased)
O'Donovan, Mrs. Marie (deceased)
Prime, Annie S. (deceased)
Sait, Eleanor L. (deceased)
Seaton, Adelaide (Mrs. A. Pearson) (deceased)
Sinclair, Jean J. (Mrs. J. Mattice) (deceased)
Thomson, Helen (Mrs. H. Harris) (deceased)

Class 1893

Anderson, Jemima A. (married) (deceased)
Bolster, Eva G. (deceased)
Bolster, Jessie (Mrs. D. N. Carmichael) (deceased)
Cave, Mary E. (deceased)
Dunlop, Jessie M. (deceased)
Hardinge, E. Hester, A.R.R.C. (deceased)
Hurcomb, Deborah J. (deceased)
Lamb, Elizabeth R. (Mrs. McLaughlin)
May, Marion M. (married)
MacDonald, Gertrude (deceased)
Morice, Lizzie (Mrs. W. D. Russell)
Pettifer, Clara (deceased)
Sullivan, Alice M. (deceased)
Sutherland, Clara L. (married)
Taylor, Annie J.
Ward, Gratia B. (Mrs. G. Spence) (deceased)

Class 1894

Barnes, Alice (married)
Beck, Florence E. (deceased)
Bickell, Elsie M. (Mrs. E. Brown) (deceased)
Bickell, M. L. (Mrs. Mabel Reid) (deceased)
Booth, Maude J. (Lady Orr-Lewis) (deceased)
Brown, Florence I. (deceased)
Boyce, Lillie (deceased)
Chipman, E. Maude (deceased)
Clouston, Bella (deceased)
Davidson, Margaret E. (deceased)
Dawson, Hilda (deceased)
DeKalb, Stella B. (Mrs. D. Patrick) (deceased)
Dodd, Ida E. (deceased)
Fortescue, Frances E. (Mrs. F. Traill) (deceased)
Fraser, Harriett (married) (deceased)
Graham, Jessie K. (deceased)
Griffen, Frances J. (deceased)
Henstchel, Matilda (Mrs. M. Jackson) (deceased)
Hersey, V. Viola (Mrs. V. Henderson) (deceased)
Lounds, Ellen S. (married)
MacPherson, Jean
McLean, Mary (married) (deceased)
Moses, Carrie E.
Ogilvie, J. M.
Phelps, Anna J. (Mrs. J. Perley)
Ross, Marion (married) (deceased)
Smith, H. M. (deceased)
Thompson, Emma (married)

Class 1895

Bullock, Agnes (deceased)
Colquhoun, Martha (deceased)
Colley, G. H. (deceased)
Hall, Frances A. (Mrs. A. Williams) (deceased)
Harper, Anna (Mrs. A. Evans) (deceased)
Lewthwaite, Sarah J. (Mrs. D. R. B. Ewan) (deceased)
LePoidevin, Mabel (Mrs. J. W. Dunfield)
Lynch, Jessie (deceased)
MacKay, Isabel (deceased)
Moffatt, Rebecca (deceased)
Ramsay, J. T. (deceased)
Smythe, Annie (Mrs. A. Taft) (deceased)
Taylor, Kate (Mrs. K. Samuel) (deceased)
Tedford, Nora (deceased)
Webster, Jennie O.B.E. (deceased)
Weston, Lyle (Mrs. L. Loucks) (deceased)

122

Class 1896

Barclay, Mrs. Annie F. (deceased)
Fair, I. Maria (deceased)
Finch, Bertha (married) (deceased)
Gilbert, Mrs. D. (deceased)
Howden, H. E.
Martin, Edith H.
McEwan, Frances D. (deceased)
McLean, Annie M. (deceased)
Munroe, Elizabeth (deceased)
Neil, Edith Ross (married)
Shaw, Flora Madeleine (deceased)
Smith, Annie (deceased)
Trenholme, Lucy H. (deceased)
Tritton, Maude (deceased)
Windel, Marguerite E.

Class 1897

Ardagh, Mrs. May
Asselstine, Carrie (deceased)
Brown, S. Ethel (deceased)
Brown, Janet F. (deceased)
Carey, Patience H. (deceased)
DesBrisay, Helen (deceased)
Dixon, Annie L.
Houghton, Grace (deceased)
MacKay, Jessie B. (Mrs. E. J. Williams) (deceased)
MacKay, Martha E. (deceased)
McLennan, Agnes M. (Mrs. A. Riopel) (deceased)
Mountain, Anabel (Mrs. A. Kerry) (deceased)
Sharp, Jessie H. (Mrs. W. Thom)
Sihler, Anna M. (married)
Sinclair, Mary E.
Smith, Mrs. Helen (deceased)
VanBuskirk, Victoria (deceased)

Class 1898

Chalmers, Lena (married) (deceased)
Evans, Beatrice A. (married) (deceased)
Franklin, Melinda C. (Mrs. M. Wainwright)
Hoerner, Sophie M., R.R.C. (Mrs. S. Price)
Lee, Ethel (deceased)
MacMillan, Bertha
McDunnough, Ethel D. (deceased)
Murdock, K. C. (deceased)
Robertson, May (Mrs. M. Shaw)
Schneider, Maude (deceased)
Spalding, Grace M.

Class 1899

Adams, Jessie (deceased)
Alcorn, Edith (Mrs. E. Burnett) (deceased)
Alexander, E. F. (married) (deceased)
Andrews, Florence (Mrs. F. L. Douglas) (deceased)
Brock, Maude (deceased)
Brown, B. W. (Mrs. J. J. Howden)
Carswell, Monica J. (married) (deceased)
Cooper, Ida S. (deceased)
Cotter, Evadne K., A.R.R.C. (deceased)
Dawson, Sarah A. (deceased)
Davis, Maude H. (deceased)
DeKalb, Ethel M. (Mrs. J. D. Webb)
Ferrier, Marie (married) (deceased)
Gallinger, Tillie (Mrs. T. Galbraith) (deceased)
Horne, Margaret L. (deceased)
Morris, Ida (deceased)
Merser, Fanny E. (deceased)
Paterson, Mary M. (deceased)
Rutledge, Edna M. (Mrs. F. M. Ball) (deceased)
Vooght, Beatrice A. (Mrs. B. A. Cook)
Watts, Mrs. K. R. (deceased)

Class 1900

Barrington, Elizabeth M. Y.
Bean, Elizabeth
Baillie, Lillie (deceased)
Binns, Effie (Mrs. E. Porter)
Brock, Kathleen (deceased)
Elder, Mary (Mrs. J. Elder) (deceased)
Fenwick, Flora (Mrs. F. McLean)
Huntley, M. Grace
Lorentz, Emma (Mrs. E. Edson) (deceased)
McGavin, Margaret (Mrs. M. Reid) (deceased)
Morton, Caroline (Mrs. W. J. Wright) (deceased)
MacMartin, L. A. (deceased)
Patton, Elizabeth (Mrs. A. J. Currie)
Quirk, Lillie (deceased)
Robinson, Mary
Russell, Florence (Mrs. F. Stevenson) (deceased)
Strumm, Flora E. (deceased)
Wainwright, Janet (deceased)
Walker, Margaret (deceased)
Young, S. F., A.R.R.C. (deceased)

Class 1901

Belknap, Frances V. (deceased)
Brook, Annie E. (Mrs. W. R. Hibbard)
Evans, Florence (Mrs. F. Sparrow) (deceased)
Gaherty, B.
Harwood, Elsie G. (Mrs. J. E. Littlehales)
(deceased)
Kennedy, Elizabeth J.
Kirkby, Florence H. (Mrs. H. H. Lyman)
(deceased)
Logie, Margaret (married)
McGee, Emily M. (Mrs. E. McGregor)
McNaughton, Barbara C. (deceased)
Ridley, Mary
Rothwell, Janet T. (Mrs. J. Dorion) (deceased)
Simpson, Kate B. (married)
Toomes, Annie
Van Zile, Mary (deceased)
Wilson, E. A. (deceased)
Wootton, S. E. (deceased)

Class 1902

Barron, Grace H. (Mrs. A. MacGregor)
Blair, Winnifred (Mrs. W. Bryce)
Daly, Georgina
Gorrell, Katherine (Mrs. K. Richardson)
Hales, Daisy
Horner, Mrs. Maude
Moore, Lillian B. (deceased)
Phipps, Ethel F.
Porteous, Dora O. (Mrs. D. Pallister)
Snowdon, Christina McF. (deceased)
Snowdon, Annie G. (deceased)
Stewart, M. Louise (deceased)

Class 1903

Addison, Sadie B.
Austin, S. (Mrs. S. Foster)
Harris, N. Elizabeth (Mrs. G. Coubrough)
Hodgins, Annie E. (married) (deceased)
Molony, Georgie M. (deceased)
Parker, M. Louise
Robinson, Bessie (deceased)
Tedford, Jessie (Mrs. J. McKay) (deceased)
Thackeray, J. W. (Mrs. J. Codere) (deceased)
Trail, Katherine (Mrs. Moodie-Heddle) (deceased)
Travers, A. M. (Mrs. A. M. Journeau)
Young, Mary Vernon (Sister Mary Virginia)

Class 1904

Armstrong, Martha J. (deceased)
Crockett, Edith S. (Mrs. Chas. Anderson)
Duncan, Jennette F. (deceased)
Edgar, Gertrude (Married) (deceased)
Fortune, Wilhelmina K. (Mrs. W. McLaughlin) (deceased)
Fraser, Sara (deceased)
Lawrence, Kate (Mrs. A. W. Blue)
Mackie, G. E. (married)
MacDonald, M. C.
McNaughton, Charlotte S. (deceased)
McCallum, Edith (Mrs. Edith Johns)
McOuat, F. D. (Mrs. Gavin Walker)
Powter, Alice G. (deceased)
Sims. J.
Sutcliffe, J. O. B. (married)
Travers, Marion (married) (deceased)
Vance, Agnes, (Mrs. J. A. Bigelow) (deceased)
Welch, Maude
Wood, Ethel H. (Mrs. W. E. Dixon) (deceased)

Class 1905

Bennett, Gertrude M. (deceased)
Blair, Cora G. (Mrs. W. A. Churchill (deceased)
Brock, Kate (deceased)
Bruce, Mary D.
Campbell, Alice E. (Mrs. R. Fraser) (deceased)
Cowen, Edith M. (deceased)
Chalmers, Helen (Mrs. H. Sare)
Fortescue, Margaret (deceased)
Howard, Evelyn
Hepburn, Mrs. Marion M. (deceased)
Malloch, A. M. (Mrs. H. S. Grindley)
McCutcheon, Ina G. (Mrs. H. R. Chillingsworth)
MacDougall, Mary
McIntosh, Alice E. (deceased)
McLeod, Lottie R. (deceased)
MacKay, Olive, A.R.R.C.
Owen, Marguerite (Mrs. Louis Andros)
Perchard, Evelyn
Ross, Elizabeth B., R.R.C. (deceased)
Shaw, Mary (Mrs. S. Barrow) (deceased)
Smardon, J. Helene (deceased)
Smith, Annie M. (Mrs. A. Connors)
Smith, Margaret I . (Mrs. Percy Simpson) (deceased)
Tough, Helen E. (Mrs. H. Nelson) (deceased)
Taylor, Marion A. (Mrs. S. W. Price)
Wells, Katherine H.
White, Lucy (deceased)
Willis, Annie T. (Mrs. A. Snyder) (deceased)

Class 1906

Anderson, Elizabeth (Mrs. Henri A. Lindsay)
Blackburn, Lillian M. M. (deceased)
Darre-Jenssen, Mrs. V.
Duncan, Flora A. (Mrs. A. Martin)
Forbes, Katherine C. (Mrs. J. MacKenzie)
Putnam, Hattie M. (Mrs. McKenzie)
Saunders, Ethel S. (Mrs. E. Chalmers) (deceased)
Vance, E. J. (Mrs. E. J. Dunbar)
White, Eleanor A. (Mrs. David Griffith)

Class 1907

Arnoldi, Christine P., A.R.R.C.
Christie, Margaret K. (Mrs. K. Murray) (deceased)
Clark, Kizzie, M. (deceased) -
Clark, K. M. MacLean (Mrs. K. Thomas)

Class 1907—Continued

Cookman, Elizabeth (Mrs. E. A. Beck)
Dow, Mrs. Lucille P. (deceased)
Hay, Jessie D.
Heron, Euphemia (deceased)
Hunter, Jean A. (Mrs. V. C. Croutch) (deceased)
Kerr, Jean
Kerr, Sara (Mrs. A. Graham)
Lane, Jennie (Mrs. Charles W. Ross) (deceased)
Malcolm, Helen C.
Maxwell, Eva (deceased)
Mitchell, Minnie A.
Sampson, Violet E. (deceased)
Swift, Eve (Mrs. John MacDermot)
Tremaine, Vivian, R.R.C. (deceased)
Trew, Eileen E.
Welch, Florence M. (deceased)
Willis, May (Mrs. W. Swift)

Class 1908

Arkison, Maude P. (Mrs. W. L. Mussell)
Clark, Muriel Birkett
Colbourn, Jennie L. (married)
Davies, Isabel, A.R.R.C.
DesBrisay, Amy S. (deceased)
Dwyer, Amy
Forbes, Mildred Hope, R.R.C. (deceased)
Hammond, Lucy B. (Mrs. Jas. Rintoul)
Hogan, Margaret (deceased)
Hutchins, Harriet (Mrs. J. Waugh) (deceased)
Ingraham, Idella M.
Law, Alice M. (Mrs. J. D. MacKerras)
Merriman, Alice M. (Mrs. McCorkindale)
McLeod, Louise F. (Mrs. Harry Cleveland)
McMurrich, Helen M., Croix de Guerre (deceased)
McRae, Mary (deceased)
Nichol, Gwendoline (deceased)
Nichol, Isabel (Mrs. James Johnston) (deceased)
Smith, Bertha A.
Upton, E. Frances, A.R.R.C. (deceased)
Wills, Edith C. (Mrs. E. Henderson) (deceased)
Wood, Rachel (deceased)

Class 1909

Barrett, Susan A.
Burnham, M. E. (deceased)
Burrows, Nancy H.
Brown, Florence W. (Mrs. G. Harper)
Brown, Winnifred
Clayton, Nellie (Mrs. A. R. Whittall) (deceased)
Campbell, Elizabeth (Mrs. L. L. Derby)
Davis, Ida M. (Mrs. I. Jacobs)
Dewar, Marion F.
Eagleson, Rosetta (Mrs. F. Rutherford) (deceased)
Gillis, L. (Mrs. B. Cumberledge)
Grahame, Janie B.
Harman, Frances A.
Haszard, Helen L. (Mrs. H. Leigh-Spencer)
Kneen, F. F. (Mrs. J. G. Anderson) (deceased)
Lovering, Mary V.
McKenzie, Georgieanna (deceased)
McTaggart, Ruth (deceased)
Nelson, Helen (Mrs. H. Robilliard) A.R.R.C. (deceased)
Palmer, Ethel R.
Reynolds, Bessie (Mrs. B. Woodburn) (deceased)
Sare, Winifred M. (Mrs. S. Redman)
Skinner, A. L.
Templeman, Carrie
Watling, Christina, A.R.R.C. (deceased)
Whitmarsh, F. Anna (Mrs. A. Brown)
Wilson, Jean G. (Mrs. J. McOuat)

Class 1910

Adams, A. H.
Barry, Mina J. (Mrs. J. Delaney) (deceased)
Betters, Pauline (Mrs. B. Hammond)
Carman, Harriet E. (deceased)
Caldwell, Winnifred H. (Mrs. H. F. Cook)
Darroch, Margaret I. (Mrs. M. Watters) (deceased)
Dickie, Lillian
Falconer, J. (Mrs. Glen Harley) (deceased)
Fowler, Jessie
French, E. (Mrs. A. S. Findlay)
Hadrill, Dorothy (deceased)
Johnston, Adelaide (Mrs. W. S. Baird)
Ketchen, Alice (deceased)
Loggie, Ruth
Templeton, M. J. (Mrs. David Fraser)
Terrill, Laura (deceased)
Walker, F. L.
Watters, Everetta (deceased)

Class 1911

Anderson, E. (Mrs. F. W. Lamb)
Anderson, Lena C. (Mrs. J. J. Ower)
Barnstead, Ethel
Batcheller, Alice H. (Mrs. A. Creighton)
Baynes, Gertrude
Beckstead, Agnes (deceased)
Caffin, Annette M. (Mrs. Farquhar Rankling)
Clark, Ethel
Day, Millicent A.
Dogherty, F. M.
Engelke, E. G.
Fraser, Lottie (Mrs. B. Burwell) (deceased)
Greetham, P. (Mrs. H. Power)
Jamieson, Agnes (deceased)
MacDermot, M. L.
MacFarlane, M. F.
McLeod, M. B. (Mrs. T. Dennison)
Read, E. L.
Read, F. M. (deceased)
Smith, Katherine M. (Mrs. K. M. Clark)
(deceased)
Smith Muriel (Mrs. Dr. Sahler)
Vipond, Gertrude (Mrs. J. W. Graham) (deceased)
Welch, M. Florence (Mrs. E. C. Renouf)
Wilson, Kate M.
Wyman, M. (Mrs. S. E. Thames)

Class 1912

Arnoldi, Gertrude (Mrs. E. Eberts) (deceased)
Brittain, Mary B. (Mrs. M. Trotter) (deceased)
Cann, Amy (Mrs. A. Nicolson) (deceased)
Carter, Lillian M. (deceased)
Cooper, A. M. (deceased)
Evans, Harriet S.
Engelke, Minnie, A.R.R.C.
Firth, Grace J. (deceased)
Gass, Clare
Gibson, Eva B. (Mrs. E. M. Smith)
Knight, Kathleen M. (deceased)
Lang, Anna E.
MacNutt, E. B.
McGreer, Louise, A.R.R.C. (deceased)
Meigs, Jessie
Moores, B. A.
Murphy, M. Anne (deceased)
Reed, Frances L. (Mrs. L. Fisher)
Scott, Susan D. (Mrs. A. A. Putnam)
Slack, Charlotte (deceased)
Stuart, Constance M. (Mrs. N. C. Stuart)
Tuck, Nellie (deceased)
Viggars, Ruth
Vipond, Grace
Wall, Rose (Mrs. Alex. McRae)

Class 1913

Armitage, Beatrice (Mrs. Howard Dixon)
Babbitt, Pearl (Mrs. Arthur Walter)
Bagshaw, Estharol (deceased)
Clark, Lillian C. (deceased)
Childs, Bessie
Cole, Marion C. (Mrs. Harris B. Todd) (deceased)
Dalgleish, Flora (Mrs. C. H. Robson)
Decou, Gertrude (Mrs. John Gale)
Elliott, Marion K. (Mrs. David Moore) (deceased)
Galt, Cecily (Mrs. John Moser) A.R.R.C.
Giffin, Mrs. Edna (deceased)
Gordon, Mrs. N. Phyllis
Gray, Lilly M., A.R.R.C.
Hart, Yvonne (Mrs. E. L. Baptist)
Handcock, Eleanor D.
Hooper, A. J. (Mrs. A. M. Leutner)
Holland, Laura, C.B.E., A.R.R.C. (deceased)
Jones, Dora H.
Lee, Winnifred A.
Leys, Cecil S. (Mrs. J. R. Oulton) (deceased)
Loggie, Rae
Muir, Marie (deceased)
O'Regan, Alice M.
Sare, Gladys I. (deceased)
Stericker, Ruth F.
Thompson, Margaret B.
Urquhart, Lottie M. M. (Mrs. Reginald W. Seys)
Whitney, Eveline M. (Mrs. E. Robbins) A.R.R.C.
(deceased)
Young, Ethel M. (Mrs. John Reid)

Class 1914

Campbell, Granger (deceased)
French, Jean (Mrs. J. Cairns)
Gordon, Winnifred (Mrs. H. Plaunt)
Gourlay, Roberta (Mrs. H. M. Powell) (deceased)
Hobkirk, Isobel (Mrs. I. Wrath) (deceased)
Kennedy, Anna G. (deceased)
Mann, J. E. (deceased)
Massy, Georgina
Morewood, Anna (deceased)
McConnell, Rachel, A.R.R.C.
McDonald, Sarah
McLeod, Katherine A., A.R.R.C.
McLennan, Hannah (Mrs. H. Fraser) (deceased)
Orr, Mrs. Mary (Mrs. M. Gough)
Pelletier, Juliette (Mrs. Stuart Ramsey)
Perry, Florence S. (Mrs. F. Labbetter)
Pettigrew, J. (Mrs. J. A. Falle)
Ross, Marjorie (deceased)
Roy, Nora (Mrs. Stanley Kirkland)
Stewart, Catherine A. (deceased)
Stevens, Myrtle
Strathy, Isabella (Mrs. A. O. McMurtry)
A.R.R.C.
Tate, Annette M., A.R.R.C.
Thomas, Annie E. (Mrs. T. H. Lennox) (deceased)
Todd, Carrie E. (Mrs. H. W. Dixon)
Whitehead, Maud (Mrs. M. Spencer)
Webb, Marjorie (Mrs. Percy Turcot) A.R.R.C.

Class 1915

Arnoldi, Helen
Babbitt, Arthura (Mrs. F. A. Beaugrand)
Barrett, Caroline V.
Caswell, Edith (Mrs. E. Hamilton)
Downes, Dorothy (Mrs. A. Gillespie)
Fishbourne, Leila
Gordon, Lillian (Mrs. Coleman Anderson)
Gullison, Beulah (Mrs. A. D. Perry)
Larter, Lily G. (Mrs. M. Bourke)
Larter, Violet (Mrs. F. L. Gribble)
Lanktree, Louise (Mrs. L. Soet)

Class 1915—Continued

Lawrence, Grace (Mrs. G. P. LeGrand) (deceased)
MacDougall, Stella
Odell, Elizabeth W., R.R.C.
Outterson, Bernice (deceased)
Patterson, Ethel M. (Mrs. C. A. Spencer)
Pyke, Helen (Mrs. H. Griffith) (deceased)
Sargeant, Agnes C.
Scott, Winnifred F. (Mrs. J. M. Jack)
Watts, Marguerite M. G. (deceased)

Class 1916

Affleck, Mildred (Mrs. M. Bryce)
Barwick, Olive (Mrs. O. Edwards) (deceased)
Briggs, Bessie E.
Clarke, Bertha (Mrs. C. Barry)
Daly, Eileen A. (Mrs. N. J. Henchey)
Dewar, E. J. (Mrs. W. M. Woodside)
Earle, G. Mildred
France, Lena (Mrs. L. Sproule)
Fuller, Florence (deceased)
Gillespie, Margaret A.
Graves, Jennie M. (deceased)
Hanley, Agnes (Mrs.
Harris, E. A. C. (Mrs. Ernest Morton)
Holland, Gertrude
Jones, M. L. (Mrs.
Kennedy, J. S.
Lester, Dell
MacArthur, Jessie (Mrs. George Hunter)
MacCallum, M. (deceased)
Macdonell, Ella (deceased)
McLeod, C. S.
McLeod, Mary W. (Mrs. M. McGregor)
May, E. J. (deceased)
Miller, Alice (Mrs. F. Downes)
Moore, Bessie C.
Motherwell, Catherine
Munro, J. F.
Paget, Gertrude (deceased)
Purdy, M. J.
Riddell, Winnifred C. (Mrs. Arthur Hunter)
Robinson, Charlotte I.
Rolland, Ethel (Mrs. E. Young)
Scarlett, Elizabeth (Mrs. E. Bradley)
Stevens, Annie J. (Mrs. R. McNutt)
Tait, Edith S. (Mrs. E. Metcalfe)
Tanner, Edith R. (Mrs. E. Kirkpatrick) (deceased)
Wales, Evelyn M.
Woods, E. (Mrs.
Wheeler, Barbara H.

Class 1917

Brissenden, L. M. (Mrs. C. K. Morrison)
Brown, M. Lewis (deceased)
Cameron, Mary S. (Mrs. K. Chisholm)
Caswell, Lillian (deceased)
Cather, Nellie M. (deceased)
Farrell, Eva M. (Mrs. E. Wilson)
Fleming, Christina (Mrs. Millar Caldwell)
Gilmour, Ethel (Mrs. W. Rogers)
Gruer, Elspeth
Hadrill, Beatrice M. (deceased)
Hogge, Ethel (Mrs. E. Learmouth)
Kenyon, Amy (Mrs. George Wood)
Livingston, Catherine (Mrs. K. Horton)
Montgomery, Mary E. H.
Moss, Dorothy (Mrs. K. Morrison) (deceased)
Murdoch, Charlotte
Murphy, Jane Alice (deceased)
McCarthy, Pauline (Mrs. A. W. Wigglesworth)
McDonald, Bertha E. (Mrs. Scott Elliott Bird)

Class 1917—Continued

McGinnis, Eva (deceased)
MacGregor, Evelyn
McIntosh, Lulu
McKay, Amy E.
Nelson, Gladys (Mrs. R. Hastings) (deceased)
Odmark, Linda J. (Mrs. L. P. House)
Peach, Elizabeth M. (Mrs. A. G. Cockrell)
Pharoah, M. M.
Reid, Annie F. (deceased)
Sharpe, Nina (Mrs. Thos. Thompson)
Smith, Jessie I.
Sowler, Elizabeth
Stewart, Nellie M.
Tracey, Helen E. (deceased)
Tracey, Lillian (deceased)
Welsh, Olive T.
Whitney, Adelaide C.

Class 1918

Brown, Nina M.
Burrell, Ida (deceased)
Clark, K. E.
Conrad, E. L.
Curwell, Nancy, (Mrs. N. Warren) (deceased)
Doré, Antoinette (Mrs. G. Elliott)
Dunwoody, Mrs. F. J.
Eaton, M. (Mrs. E. MacNeily)
Elmslie, Olive
Ewing, G. I. (Mrs. R. Cooke)
Farmer, Shirley (Mrs. G. Baptist) (deceased)
Gifford, D. (Mrs. D. Goodrich)
Gray, Irene (Mrs. C. A. Marlatt)
Gray, M., Q.A.I.M.S.S.
Harland, M.
Heeschen, M. (Mrs. H. B. Church) (deceased)
Home, Jean
Keirstead, Mrs. Hazel E.
Lightbound, M. (Mrs. M. Devine)
Little, Ethelwyn (Mrs. E. Vargo)
Lowery, M. V.
McCammon, M. A. (Mrs. J. T. Allan)
McKinnon, Lillian F.
Nichols, R.
Rhodes, D. (Mrs. T. A. Evans)
Robbins, L. (Mrs. Lionel Whitehead)
Ross, Amy M.
Ross, H. M.
Sinton, M. (Mrs. N. J. Ferguson)
Smith, A. B.
Stewart, L. (Mrs. W. B. Scott)
Walsh, Jane (deceased)
Willett, B. (Mrs. G. McLelland)
Willis, Margaret (deceased)
Wyman, Emma

Class 1919

Adams, Alma (Mrs. A. Foley)
Aubrey, Gertrude (Mrs. F. W. Tetley) (deceased)
Aubrey, Tessie (Mrs. Morley Holland)
Allison, R. G. (Mrs. H. B. Ainsley)
Adair, Lilian (Mrs. C. C. Stewart)
Belyea, Mrs. Myrtle
Bennets, Marjorie
Blenkinsop, H. L.
Boa, Marion
Brackenbusch, E. M. (Mrs. F. Kolesch)
Calder, Gertrude M.
Estey, Hazel A. (Mrs. A. Pflatz)
Fox, Miriam R. (Mrs. L. Young)
Foxall, F. E. (Mrs. E. E. Wellington)
Fraser, Lillian

Class 1919—Continued

Henderson, Edna L. (Mrs. E. Atkinson)
Holt, Mabel K.
Hyndman, L. S. (Mrs. L. Moulton)
Ketchen, A. G. (Mrs. O. Ellis)
Laing, C. M. (Mrs. C. Merson)
Lambart, C. A. (deceased)
Leonowens, Anna (Mrs. A. H. L. Monahan)
Lindsay, Edythe
Lomer, E. M. (Mrs. W. Telford)
Matheson, Florinda M.
Merkley, Ida B.
Moody, Marjorie B. (Mrs. C. B. Leggo)
Morell, Janet L.
Macfie, Annie M.
Peters, Mary (Mrs. F. R. Fraser)
Pincock, Nellie (Mrs.
Scott, Winnifred (Mrs. W. Beavis)
Sampson, Audrey, (Mrs. John Calder)
Seveigny, Elsa C. (Mrs. H. D. Caswell)
Smith, K. (Mrs. A. O. Allan) (deceased)
Skelton, Mrs. Emily
Shaw, Helen B. (deceased)
Stack, Hannah M. (Mrs. Glen Roberts)
Symonds, Isabel
Townsend, Helene
Vaudry, Mrs. Pearl (Mrs. R. Ruel)
Venne, Stella M. (deceased)
Tulloch, Elsie M. (deceased)

Class 1920

Alcombrack, Frances (Mrs. A. L. Windsor)
Ayling, Elizabeth (Mrs. E. Bromley)
Armstrong, Ferol (Mrs. J. Ward)
Barclay, Annie (Mrs. R. H. Brown)
Belyea, Annie (Mrs. G. Warren)
Bruce, Dorothea (Mrs. D. McRae)
Buchanan, Mildred
Carroll, Pauline (Mrs. H. C. Hickey)
Davis, Caroline (Mrs. B. MacLean)
Denovan, Christina
Dulmadge, Catherine (Mrs. W. M. Redmond)
Duncan, Mary (Mrs. H. T. Mitchell)
Ewing, Isabel (Mrs. R. V. Russell)
Faulkner, Katherine
Goldie, Marjorie (Mrs. N. Noseworthy)
Golding, Maude
Haines, Lila
Jackson, Marguerite
Jamieson, Eva (Mrs. J. A. Upham)
Jessiman, Phyllis
Johnston, Mary
Little, Bertha (Mrs. J. B. Eveleigh)
Long, Mary (deceased)
McNabb, Janet (Mrs. J. J. Higgins)
McIntosh, C. McK. (Mrs. A. V. Hardwick)
Morrison, Margaret (Mrs. Fred Cole)
Parsons, Emily
Parks, Hattie (Mrs. H. J. Wayne)
Peters, Helen (deceased)
Ramsay, Mrs. Gladys (deceased)
Sinton, B. A.
Sproule, Eva
Strople, Eva
Taylor, Isabel
Taylor, Irene (Mrs. A. E. Rowlands)
Thompson, Flora (deceased)
Vizard, Jean
Wallace, Dorothy (Mrs. F. J. Cunningham)
Wells, Beatrice (Mrs. B. Moss) (deceased)
Wilcox, Celia
Young, Gladys (deceased)
Young, Mabel (deceased)

Class 1921

Alford, Hazel
Allward, Annie
Allward, Vera
Batson, Martha (deceased)
Beck, Edna (Mrs. J. Lyons)
Brewster, Alice
Brinton, Beatrice (Mrs. John Newman) (deceased)
Budden, Janie (Mrs. G. W. Crombie)
Clarke, Frances
Elliott, Helen
Gardiner, Winifred
Gunning, Ione (Mrs. Arthur Rowan)
Hewton, Helen
Higgins, Melba (Mrs. James Baker)
Hodge, Florence (Mrs. J. Breckinridge)
Hunt, Fern (Mrs. Fern H. Lusk)
Jackson, Gertrude (Mrs. G. Keep) (deceased)
Jamieson, Janie
Johns, Edna (Mrs. James Rowlings)
King, Kathleen (Mrs. A. Parkinson)
MacKay, Anna (Mrs. E. Lyons) (deceased)
MacMillan, Mattie (Mrs. B. Black)
MacDermot, Dorothea
McGrand, Sadie
Mann, Louise (Mrs. C. Clements)
Martin, Marion E.
Milton, Susan (deceased)
Ross, Marjorie (Mrs. J. Wathen)
Smith, Winnifred (Mrs. T. Whittles)
Whitney, Freda

Class 1922

Aird, Libbie (Mrs. W. K. Rutherford)
Barnes, Edna (Mrs. D. L. Stewart)
Bertrand, Mrs. Eva (deceased)
Bowen, Shirley (Mrs. Esmond McWood)
Bradley, Mrs. Helen
Bullis, Dorothy (Mrs. J. Scott Williams)
Buss, Marie (Mrs. Andrew Bonnet)
Chisholm, Jean (Mrs. George Milne)
Codere, Margaret (Mrs. M. McManus)
Cooke, Gertrude (Mrs. C. S. Fosbery)
Dovey, Gertrude (Mrs. A. F. Marsh)
Dunlop, Jessie
Dutton, Edith (Mrs. Jack Street)
Gardiner, Mrs. Claudia (Mrs. C. Holling)
(deceased)
Gibbons, Marie
Hill, Muriel (Mrs. N. D. Cass)
Jackson, Clara
Journeay, Eleanor (Mrs. L. Rudolphe)
Kelly, Ina (Mrs. Bert Green) (deceased)
Lathe, Dema (Mrs. Thomas VanVliet)
Leslie, Irene (Mrs. L. R. MacDonald)
Lineham, Minnie (Mrs. A. Dutton)
Lockhart, Vivian (Mrs. V. Mason)
MacDonald, S. Marjorie
MacKay, Christina (Mrs. H. Marshall)
MacKay, E. Grace
McNeil, Francesca (Mrs. Wm. Black)
Markham, Irene
Middleton, Margaret M.
McCrea, Clara (Mrs. H. Brown)
Miller, Hazel (Mrs. C. Cutler)
Murphy, Agnes M.
Preston, Beatrice (Mrs. E. C. Menzies)
Powers, Evelyn
Ross, Lillian (Mrs. J. S. Moore)
Ross, Stella (Mrs. M. S. Hamilton)
Seaman, Annie
Scott, Madeline (Mrs. G. Williams) (deceased)
Van Vliet, Jean

127

Class 1923

Baldrey, Madge, (Mrs. C. B. Foster)
Bennett, Myrtle (Mrs. C. S. Rankin)
Brown, Isabella
Budd, Carmen (Mrs. N. MacFarlane)
Cluff, Florence (Mrs. R. S. McEachen)
DesBarres, Marie
DeVere, Tillie
Dwane, Emily (deceased)
Foster, Ruth O'Day (Mrs. Thomas Hardy)
Grandmaison, Evelyn (Mrs. R. Turcotte)
Howlett, Nina
Hutt, Anna M.
Kell, Mary M. (Mrs. E. P. Eustace)
Lawrence, Margaret
Little, Hilda
Low, Elizabeth
MacTier, Adeline (Mrs. Donald White)
McConachie, Grace (Mrs. Hodder Stovel)
McCarogher, Dorothea
McCuaig, Helena C.
MacKenzie, Katherine (Mrs. E. T. Wyman)
McCollum, Muriel (Mrs. Hugh Harding)
McLeod, Anna M. (Mrs. W. Scott)
MacRae, Mary J.
Morewood, Isabel G.
Parham, Gladys (Mrs. J. Parham)
Park, Mary O.
Parmenter, Helen (Mrs. Pierre Amos)
Prince, M. K. (Mrs. P. Herring)
Robertson, Elizabeth
Russell, Marguerite (Mrs. J. H. McCulloch)
Saucier, Violet (Mrs. Harold LeBlanc)
Shaver, Matilda M.
Shipman, Ivy (deceased)
Smellie, Estelle S. (Mrs. R. McLeod)
Smith, Jean M.
Sullivan, Eileen (Mrs. J. F. Brown)
Ward, Edythe
Welling, Inez
Whelpley, Marjorie (Mrs. G. H. Sonne)

Class 1924

Burns, Margaret (Mrs. T. Lambert)
Buzzell, Gladys
Cooke, Winnifred
Cowie, Margaret
Currie, Ina (Mrs. Arthur Manson)
Currie, Margaret J. (Mrs. F. G. Bird) (deceased)
Elliott. Hattie B. (Mrs. C. B. Black)
Frappied, Mildred (Mrs. M. Wallis)
Fraser, Audrey (Mrs. P. O'Shaughnessy)
Goode, Winnifred (Mrs. C. C. Fraser)
Heney, Ida (Mrs. E. L. Johnson)
Henderson, Ida
Hogge, Annie (Mrs. E. R. Jones)
Ives, Marian
Kelly, Jean (Mrs. N. Noseworthy)
Kirby, Elsie E.
LaCarte, Florida (deceased)
Laskey, Kathleen
LeFrancois, Elsie M. (Mrs. Harvey E. Malcom)
LeGallais, A. E. (deceased)
Montgomery, Elsie (Mrs. E. J. Price)
Morash, Mona (Mrs. A. Marryat) (deceased)
McRae, Mabel (Mrs. M. Carr)
Pollock, Elizabeth (Mrs. R. Harvey)
Riddell, Lena
Steele, Clara (Mrs. G. Fessenden) (deceased)
Stewart, Julina (Mrs. A. Neate)
Stinson, Lillian (Mrs. L. Schram)
Snow, Pearl (Mrs. B. Phillips)
Sweanor, Eleanor
Talbot, Elsie
Tanner, Grace

Class 1924—Continued

Taylor, Madeline
Whitley, Dorothy (Mrs. K. M. Heard)
Yould, Mrs. Abbie (deceased)

Class 1925

Alford. Olive L. (Mrs. J. McCulloch) (deceased)
Alshorne, Mrs. Maude
Carten, Edith (Mrs. Russell Spafford)
Carter, Grace S.
Cromwell, Anne E.
Dobbie, M. Grace (Mrs. M. G. Gilles)
Edgar, Olive (deceased)
Ewing, Grace E. (Mrs. G. Dorman)
Feeney, Marie (Mrs. M. Cain)
Fowler, Jean (Mrs. R. Herman)
Giroux, Laura (Mrs. Geo. R. Newman)
Hamilton, M. Evelyn
Hamilton, A. Ruth
Herman, Blanche G.
Horsfall, Evelyn K.
Ladd, Catherine (Mrs. R. Powell)
Labelle, Gertrude (Mrs. M. Grondin)
Lewis, Esther E. (Mrs. K. Battley)
Lunan, Isabel M.
Mathewson, Mary S. (deceased)
Mitchell, Olive A. (Mrs. A. Williams) (deceased)
Mitchell, Gladys (Mrs. Randolph Hinch)
                                    (deceased)
Mulligan, Olive
McLeod, Edith M. (Mrs. G. Murray)
MacQuisten. Edith A. (Mrs. J. Martin)
McConnell, Isabel
McCulloch, Jeanie (deceased)
McQuade, Irene (deceased)
Nicol, Lenore
Pennington, Phyllis (Mrs. Murray Stalker)
Raeburn, Margaret (Mrs. Ira J. Patton)
Shaver, Winnifred R.
Shaw, Margaret (deceased)
Smith, Gladys H. (Mrs. W. B. Holmes)
Smith, M. Hoffman (Mrs. K. A. Stewart)
Stewart, Geraldine P.
Stewart, Helen N. (deceased)
Stewart, Lucretia E.
Tanner, Hattie P.
Veira, Doris M. (Sister Raymond Mary)
Wilson, Alice B.

Class 1926

Ahern, Ethel M.
Backman, Myra (Mrs. J. F. Masterton) (deceased)
Belford, Garner (Mrs. R. Annable)
Bieber, Marjorie
Branscombe, Kathleen (Mrs. E. S. Davis)
Brown, Enid L.
Carpenter, Lily M.
Carter, Almeda (Mrs. M. G. Evans)
Christie, Marguerite (Mrs. M. Porter) (deceased)
Cole, Christine
Cromwell, Freda E. (Mrs. R. Moore)
Depew, Belle (Mrs. E. C. Armstrong)
French, Lowten
Frith, Hazel E. (Mrs. H. Malcolm)
Gaskin, Mona E. (Mrs. E. J. Opal)
Harris, Martha A. (Mrs. W. Sumner)
Harvey, Hilda (Mrs. C. Wellington)
Jones, Dorothy (Mrs. W. J. Marshall)
Jowsey, Anna Mae
Knollin, Victoria
LeQuesne, Drusee (Mrs. G. Claset)
Lewis, Doris (Mrs. N. C. Smart)
Lockwood, Edith L. (Mrs. A. Kendall)
Mercer, Miriam (deceased)
Miller, Bernice (Mrs. R. E. Horncastle)

128

Class 1926—Continued

Muir, Jean McD. (Mrs. F. Eveleigh)
Murphy, Isobel M.
Myers, Marion S.
Mackenzie, Norena A. (deceased)
MacLeod, Jennie M. (Mrs. D. MacDonald)
MacLeod, Marguerite
McCosh, Juana H.
O'Hara, Louise
Payne, Sadie M. (Mrs. Cecil Turner) (deceased)
Small, Catherine (Mrs. E. Wurtele)
Taylor, Margaret E. (Mrs. H. Johnston)
Urquhart, Donalda
Wathen, Bessie (Mrs. Ray Holmes)
Yardley, Barbara

Class 1927

Allworth, Helene (Mrs. Harold G. Pearson)
Baird, Ethel (Mrs. Gay Judson)
Barclay, Elizabeth (Mrs. H. Minhinnick)
Bateson, Lilly (Mrs. H. S. Mitchell)
Best, Lolita (Mrs. Edward Shead)
Blacklock, Grace
Brady, Katherine (Mrs. H. M. Stevenson)
Bradley, Jane
Brewster, Dorothy (Mrs. Louis Brais)
Bresee, Jessie (Mrs. J. Jackson)
Brown, Helen (Mrs. J. J. Walker)
Brown, Pauline
Byrne, Kathleen
Charland, Loretta (Mrs. J. D. Simpson) (deceased)
Coolican, Hazel (Mrs. E. N. Irvin)
Cooper, Marjorie (Mrs. H. J. Lindsay)
Cox, Isabel (Mrs. R. H. Anderson)
Donaldson, Jean (Mrs. Gordon Stroud)
Driffield, Dorothy (Mrs. R. H. Bishop)
Duggan, Noreen (Mrs. D. T. Anderson)
Duprey, Beatrice (Mrs. K. J. Kilgour)
Farmer, Frances
Forbes, Carrie
Gillies, Margaret (Mrs. C. Johnson)
Gordon, Florence (deceased)
Hart, Ethel M.
Haselton, Helen
Hayes, Janie M. (Mrs. Angus Croft)
Hill, Vivian (Mrs. C. Schroeder)
Johnston, Mrs. Hildred
Judson, Doris (Mrs. Harry Pierce)
Kenehan, Patricia M. (Mrs. P. Maloney)
(deceased)
Kirkham, Winnifred (Mrs. Stanley Hutchinson)
LeBlanc, Anna Marie (Mrs. Edward Christison)
MacDonald, Martha A.
MacGibbon, Viola (Mrs. L. Burton)
MacIsaac, Sadie
MacLeod, Vera B. (Mrs. P. Butler)
MacNeil, Jean
MacRae, Dorothy (Mrs. W. P. Warner)
McGaughey, M. Kathleen (Mrs. Edward
Martineau) (deceased)
MacKenzie, C. Hazel
McMann, Isabel M. (Mrs. John Hope)
Miller, Marion R. (Mrs. Evan Shute)
Moroney, Flora
Roberts, Emily (Mrs. E. A. S. King)
Russell, May G. (Mrs. J. McCarthy)
Seifert, Dorothy J.
Slack, Dorothy (Mrs. C. W. Fullerton)
Smith, Ida
Smith, Elizabeth (Mrs. E. A. Parry)
Sullivan, Viola (Mrs. George Dewar)
Thom, Janet M.
Thorpe, Anne
Tremaine, Phyllis (Mrs. W. A. Matthews)
Wetmore, A. Grace (Mrs. R. Johnson) (deceased)
Wims, Jessie (Mrs. John Allen)

Class 1928

Adams, F. C.
Allport, Jessie
Anderson, N. J.
Annesley, K. L. (Mrs. H. Hodkinson)
Barraclough, C. (Mrs. George Day)
Bashaw, K. Jean (Mrs. F. Adams)
Brown, A. M. (Mrs. T. B. Wainwright)
Bryson, J. H. (Mrs. Douglas Sproule)
Campbell, M. C. (Mrs. K. Mullins)
Campbell, B. L.
Church, E. L. (Mrs. T. E. Roy)
Clark, H. M.
Coffrin, D. R.
Cooke, E. B.
Cravath, M. G. (Mrs. Howard Elliott)
Davidson, D. A. (Mrs. D. Smith)
Dever, E. F.
Downs, D. M. (Mrs. G. Joseph)
Elliott, E. S. (deceased)
Foss, L. A. (Mrs. J. Copeland)
Fraser, S. (Mrs. C. B. Wright)
Grant, A. C.
Green, S. M.
Hervey, M. J. (Mrs. G. Evans)
Heisler, M. B. (Mrs. M. Burleigh)
Hessell, G. V. (Mrs. V. Kyle)
Hicks, S. A.
Hollenbeck, M. H. N.
Johnson, A. P.
Lafleur, D. M.
Lafleur, G. M.
Meggitt, M. M. (deceased)
Mills, C. W. (Mrs. A. McCormick)
Moore, E. C. (Mrs. Wm. Hogg)
Moseley, G. J. (Mrs. G. Brice)
Monk, M. (Mrs. A. Langen)
McColgan, M. G.
McLaren, A. M. (Mrs. George Hamilton)
O'Connor, S. G.
Pibus, E. M.
Percival, E. I. (Mrs. John LeMee)
Raeburn, M. J. (Mrs. John Stewart)
Seaman, B. M.
Simpson, R. A. (Mrs. E. M. Hill)
Shaver, L. E. (Mrs. R. deBoyrie)
Shepherd, D. W. (Mrs. D. Saxton)
Shepherd, L. M. (deceased)
Smeaton, G. A.
Smith, F. E. M. (Mrs. A. S. Turnbull)
Stephenson, D. R. (Mrs. Guy M. Wynn)
Sterling, E. G.
Stewart, A. (Mrs. A. Russell)
Sutherland, Jean (Mrs. C. T. M. McClellan)
Swan, M. A. (Mrs. E. W. Harding) (deceased)
Turner, K. A.
Vass, G. M. (Mrs. G. A. McHardy)
Wells, A. I.

Class 1929

Adams, Ottilie (Mrs. Norman Cameron)
Adams, Florence (Mrs. G. Henderson)
Buchanan, Agnes V. (Mrs. A. Blenkinship)
Butler, R. E. (Mrs. W. Wright)
Campbell, Margaret (Mrs. W. E. Gillespie)
Chisholm, Beryl M. (Mrs. Leslie Howlett)
Coleman, Frances E.
Conrad, Christina A. (Mrs. Maurice Carew)
Cregeen, Elsie
Cruise, Mary A. (Mrs. Allen Muir)
Cutter, Eva L.
Denniston, Margaret
Dunlop, Jean M. (Mrs. Gordon Ladd)
Fletcher, Alma
Flint, Dorothy
Gilmour, Leslie L.

Class 1929—Continued

Gustafson, Pauline (Mrs. H. M. Belton)
Hawley, Glenna (Mrs. Gordon Caple)
Henrikson, Elie M. (Mrs. E. M. Wright)
Imrie, Margaret F. (Mrs. M. S. Lothrop)
Johnston, Melba E.
Kearns, Catherine (Mrs. H. Hamilton)
Kent, Bernice
Lamb, Frances M. (Mrs. R. D. Towle)
Lamb, Ivy M. (Mrs. V. G. Streadwick)
Lamplough, Isobel (Mrs. T. L. Overing)
Lennon, Agnes F. (Mrs. F. J. Woodall)
Macklaier, Dorothy M. (Mrs. J. A. Gauthier)
Mallalieu, Iris C. (deceased)
McBride, Marjorie J. (Mrs. J. Thomlinson)
MacDonald, Theodora
MacKay, Margaret (Mrs. E. McCourt)
MacQueen, Isobel (Mrs. Gordon Scott)
McMaster, Grace K. (Mrs. Harold Webster)
MacVean, Martha A. (Mrs. J. S. Arbuckle)
Newton, Margaret D. (Mrs. R. M. Snowdon)
Noble, Barbara G. (Mrs. M. M. Ross)
Perry, Grace A. (Mrs. G. LeBaron)
Porteous, Kathleen (deceased)
Rogers, Aileen E.
Kennedy-Reid, Nancy B.
Schonnop, Helen (deceased)
Seymour, Daisy B. (Mrs. S. Rogers)
Shepherd, Helen M.
Shields, Ina (Mrs. Chester Woodbine)
Smith, Anna Mae (Mrs. S. M. Banfill) (deceased)
Staple, Myrtle L. (Mrs. J. Petite)
Taylor, Marjorie L. (Mrs. C. A. Woodside)
Whyte, Evelyn I. (Mrs. Arch. MacDonald)

Class 1930

Ainslie, J. E.
Baker, A. E.
Barry, G. A. (Mrs. S. S. Joule)
Brady, M. L. E. (Mrs. M. Thornton)
Brokenshire, H. A.
Campbell, F. E. (Mrs. F. W. Snell)
Cass, H. S. (Mrs. S. B. Fraser)
Clancy, V. E.
Cook, M. I. (Mrs. F. R. Crumbie)
Dea, C. A. (Mrs. John Aylen)
Doherty, M. E. (Mrs. R. Buchanan)
Draper, M. E. (Mrs. F. Calder)
Eaman, G. L. (Mrs. G. L. Udd)
Fischer, E. H. (Mrs. J. R. Parmley)
Gould, F. E. (Mrs. C. B. Neapole)
Hansen, N. H. (Mrs. B. G. Hamilton) (deceased)
Higgins, D. V. (Mrs. W. R. McGlaughlin)
Hunter, M. E.
King, W. E.
Knox-Wight, B. M. (Mrs. B. M. Page) (deceased)
Lumbers, M. J. (deceased)
Martin, S. I. (Mrs. Lloyd Powell)
Manley, C. H. (Mrs. R. G. Sampson)
Messenger, K. (Mrs. Clarence Miller) (deceased)
Mignot, D. I. (Mrs. E. H. Ingalls)
Miller, I. M. (Mrs. Stanley Adlam) (deceased)
Mitchell, F. I. (Mrs. I. Rice)
Moses, M. (Mrs. H. Warren)
McCarron, C. G. (Mrs. T. Reilley)
MacDonald, C. F. (Mrs. C. F. Bambrick)
MacDonald, J. W. (Mrs. W. A. Eskil)
MacDonald, J. E. (Mrs. J. A. Casey)
MacDonald, Rebecca
McLaren, J. M. (Mrs. J. Crosbie) (deceased)
MacLeod, M. I.
Norris, C. A.
Orman, M. A. (Mrs. L. Bishop)
Parker, I. L. (Mrs. Philip Rowe)
Pearson, H. (Mrs. E. Reid)
Pritchard, S. H. (Mrs. C. L. F. Watchorn)

Class 1930—Continued

Randall, F. E. (Mrs. K. W. Fraser)
Reid, A. G.
Reid, E. S.
Robicheau, E. M. (Mrs. D. Byers)
Robinson, M. E. (Mrs. Jules Bertrand) (deceased)
Ruse, C. J. (Mrs. J. Meagher)
Shaw, H. D.
Snow, D. T. (Mrs. E. B. Anderson)
Spier, H. W. (deceased)
Smith, A. B. (Mrs. L. Seldon)
Smith, B. J. (Mrs. R. A. Wight)
Stedman, Louise (deceased)
Sutherland, A. M. (Mrs. R. G. Quinlan)
Turnbull, E. M. (Mrs. T. Bagley)
Wallace, M. (Mrs. J. S. MacNeish)
Welling, H.
Willis, Lyle D. (deceased)
Winsor, E. M. (Mrs. G. Brownrigg)
Wootton, J. E. (Mrs. F. J. Mahaffy)
Wright, F. H.

Class 1931

Aitkenhead, C. B.
Baird, L. M. B.
Bartsch, H. M. (deceased)
Bedore, M. (Mrs. John Berg)
Bergeron, M. J. (Mrs. Eric Hopwood)
Boucher, Y. M. (Mrs. Yvonne Adams)
Cameron, R. F.
Candlish, R. C. (Mrs. H. Lester)
Chisholm, L. K. (Mrs. E. deLalla)
Currie, G. A. (deceased)
Doyle, E. (Mrs. E. D. Maher)
Dunn, Clara (Mrs. J. T. Shane)
Elder, H. E. (Mrs. Percy Marsden)
Elford, F. M.
Falconer, H. E. (Mrs. J. W. Levy)
Falls, R. S.
Flatt, S. A. (Mrs. J. Warmington)
Franckum, B. G.
French, F. (Mrs. F. Small)
Gardner, H. M. (Mrs. H. Digby-Leigh)
Gibson, J. Z. (Mrs. George Dempster) (deceased)
Goodfellow, A. F. (Mrs. J. Bushe)
Graham, V. (Mrs. R. Wallingford)
Grant, A. (Mrs. A. Guillet)
Haselton, W. I. (Mrs. T. Tyson)
Hass, A. B. (Mrs. A. Tsikaris)
Hennessey, M. C. (Mrs. Ian Balmar)
Hillary, B. S. (Mrs. L. J. Adams)
Holtby, D. (Mrs. G. R. Cullen)
Howard, M. A. (Mrs. M. A. Kenwood)
Hughes, E. M. (Mrs. E. H. Murphy)
Hume, A. G. (Mrs. Jack Gunn)
Hunting, G. I. (Mrs. A. Hunting)
Irving, H. G.
Jousse, E. M. (Mrs. T. C. Walcot)
Kavanagh, E. A. (Mrs. T. J. Rowan)
King, E. M. R. (Mrs. H. W. Capel)
Levie, M. (Mrs. J. Demers)
Lilley, O. H.
Martin, G. B. (Mrs. K. A. Sheltus)
Mifflin, M. E. (Mrs. G. Carson)
Morgan, D. M. (Mrs. Rupert Holland)
Morrison, I. K. (Mrs. James Davison)
Mugridge, J. E. (Mrs. F. B. Tilton)
Murphy, D. E.
MacDonald, C. M. (Mrs. E. A. MacNaughton)
MacMillan, M. S. (Mrs. Michael McMullen)
MacMurchy, B. M.
McArthur, F. E. (Mrs. James McCoy)
McCarthy, M. M. (Mrs. A. T. Jousse)
McLean, M. M. (Mrs. H. B. Olsen) (deceased)
McLennan, E. S. (Mrs. E. S. Dae)
McRae, J. B. (Mrs. Jack Dingwall)
Neil, G. I. (Mrs. J. R. Bartlett)

Class 1931—Continued

Philips, R. E. (Mrs. Henry Williams)
Pounden, M. G. (Mrs. H. Johnson) (deceased)
Rogers, S. E. (Mrs. S. Pearson)
Ross, M. (Mrs.) (Mrs. M. L. Manley)
Savard, J. M. E. (Mrs. R. A. Lombard)
Sharpe, L. F.
Smith, E. I. (Mrs. E. Peters)
Smith, M. G. (Mrs. J. Sanbourne)
Steele, F. W. (Mrs. George Watchorn)
Watson, H. I. (Mrs. F. Garrison)
Webber, H. V. (Mrs. L. Thayer)
Welling, D. M. (Mrs. E. Carlson)
Wilson, A. M. (Mrs. W. H. Boyd)
Woolner, M. L. (Mrs. F. Hockin)
Wren, L. D.
Yelland, May (Mrs. M. Hendry)
Yule, K. C. (Mrs. C. Johnston)

Class 1932

Almond, V. B.
Anderson, C. L. (Mrs. Stuart Townsend)
Baxter, M. A. (Mrs. Fergus Johnston)
Bernard, M. E. (Mrs. Gilbert Beatty)
Blakney, G. E. (Mrs. Henry Drew)
Bradford, E. M.
Brewer, A. G. (Mrs. Albert Gillespie)
Campbell, E. E. (Mrs. H. Wilson)
Christie, N. T. (deceased)
Coffin, E. M. (Mrs. C. Dakin)
Copland, M. G. (Mrs. Leon Sanborne)
Cosman, D. L. (Mrs. C. A. Bradley)
Coughtry, A. F. (Mrs. D. McMillan)
Crandell, M. F.
Denman, E. I.
Donald, E. (Mrs. Clarence Tryon)
Dustin, J. P. (deceased)
Evans, F. (Mrs. Eric Tutching)
Fish, E. M. (Mrs. R. Stewart)
Foster, C. H. (Mrs. N. Schindler)
Frizzell, I. A. (Mrs. Donald Chisholm)
Fulton, M. E. (Mrs. Wm. Fair)
Gemeroy, I. F. (Mrs. Isabelle Keyes)
Goobie, P. M. (Mrs. B. Daniels)
Hamilton, M. C. (Mrs. W. Gibson)
Harvey, A. J. (Mrs. D. B. Patterson)
Henstridge, M. K. (Mrs. N. Stewart)
Hjertholm, G. P. (Mrs. G. Highland)
King, J. E. (Mrs. E. W. Pickard) (deceased)
Lockhart, H. P. (Mrs. John MacLean)
Marshall, E. R. (Mrs. A. B. Rilance)
Maynes, E. M. (Mrs. O. Lewis)
Meighen, Norah L.
Melkman, F. E. (Mrs. Allan Von Blerk)
Michaels, Carol (Mrs. J. Friedman)
Michaud, Y. (Mrs. F. J. Leger)
Moffatt, E. W. (Mrs. E. McAlpine)
Murphy, A. M. (Mrs. F. Francis)
Murphy, M. deS. (Mrs. Bernard Watson)
McIver, Isobel (Mrs. G. H. Logie)
MacKinnon, F. M. (Mrs. James Forrest)
MacLeod, K. C.
MacRae, V. M.
McCracken, D. M. (Mrs. H. H. Skelton)
McKiel, M. E. (Mrs. T. O. Evans)
Osmond, K. S.
Petrie, D. S. (Mrs. Ralph McIntosh)
Rodger, A. B.
Roe, O. M. (Mrs. Ross Bowes)
Shannon, M. A.
Shaw, H. K.
Small, M. E.
Sprigings, C. B. (Mrs. Kenneth Monks)
Steele, B. E. (Mrs. H. J. Hooper)
Sykes, E. M.
Underhill, B. C.

Class 1932—Continued

Watson, E. H. (Mrs. Lloyd Somerville)
Wilbur, M. K. (Mrs. Edwin Steeves)
Wilson, O. H.
Wolstenholme, D. E.

Class 1933

Almond, M. J. (Mrs. W. S. Bouillon)
Bassett, L. W.
Boyd, E. M. (Mrs. Jackson Crawford)
Bradshaw, H. W.
Burri, L. M. (Mrs. Alex. Cowan)
Cadegan, M. C.
Colquhoun, D. R.
Cooke, M. E. (Mrs. C. G. Rowe)
Coombs, E. M. (Mrs. B. Grime)
Davy, Enid
Dougall, L. N. (Mrs. J. F. Blue)
Dundin, M. V. (Mrs. M. Sullivan)
Dunn, M. V.
Dunn, S. I. (deceased)
Fischer, F. J. (Mrs. C. W. Adams)
Fitzgerald, C. (Mrs. Morley McKelvey)
Flewelling, M. E. (Mrs. W. M. MacLean)
Foote, M. K. (Mrs. C. Honey)
Gilbert, I. M. (Mrs. R. Randall)
Grant, H. B. (Mrs. A. J. Tyler) (deceased)
Grist, T. A.
Hamilton, H. G.
Hardy, G. H. (Mrs. G. English)
Jackson, C. M. (Mrs. Earl Radley)
King, H. H. (Mrs. H. Featherstone)
Lamb, Rosamond
Lamont, M. E. (Mrs. W. A. Martinson)
Leslie, B. L.
LeTemplier, F.
Michie, D. L.
Miller, M. (deceased)
Moss, B. (Mrs. T. S. Johnstone)
MacDonald, R. A. (Mrs. G. R. Rinfret)
MacLeod, K. M. (Mrs. Fred MacKenzie)
McConnell, G. I. (Mrs. Leonard Carroll)
McKenzie, J. R.
McKim, K. S.
McQueen, M. E. (Mrs. G. D. Madison)
Peverley, Ann
Piette, G. T.
Quinn, L. M. (Mrs. John McGill)
Ramey, C. N.
Rollitt, H. (Mrs. H. Crompton)
Scott, V. A. (Mrs. W. H. Smith)
Siddons-Gray, N.
Smith, M. M. (Mrs. J. E. Morrison)
Stoot, B.
Tanner, I. M. (Mrs. P. F. Bell)
Titcomb, L. E. (Mrs. J. F. McGill)
Turner, C. W.
Warwick, M. (Mrs. J. J. Miller)
Wylie, B. A. (Mrs. L. Wylie)

Class 1934

Armstrong, G. P. (Mrs. Hurd F. Reynolds)
Atkinson, M. (Mrs. D. de la Roche)
Belford, Nora (Mrs. Arthur Silver)
Blandford, V. R. (Mrs. G. German)
Bonner, D. I. (Mrs. G. Wood)
Campbell, A. M. (Mrs. P. Conway)
Cerat, M. A.
Eaves, B. A. (Mrs. C. Barker)
Fernie, D. F. (Mrs. L. D. Gardner)
Fulton, H. E. M. (Mrs. R. Scanlon)
Graham, B. M.
Hall, E. M. (deceased)
Higman, P. E. (Mrs. Roy McDougall)
Hiscocks, C. (Mrs. Lawrence Govan)

131

Class 1934—Continued

Hobson, D. I. (Mrs. J. P. Landon)
Irving, M. A.
King, E. P. (Mrs. T. E. Bennett)
Latta, M. I.
Legere, H. D. (Mrs. J. B. MacDonald)
Linklater, M. M. (Mrs. L. C. Haslam)
McGillivray, S. J. (Mrs. Harvey Jack)
McKean, M. E. (Mrs. P. D. Baird)
MacLean, G. H. (Mrs. D. A. Johnson)
Melanson, A. M. (Mrs. L. K. Coffin)
Mercer, A. G. (Mrs. H. Sharpe)
Miller, H. J. (Mrs. Alan Taylor)
Neilson, W. D. L. (Mrs. Guy Moreau)
Pope, M. A. (Mrs. J. B. Poole)
Porter, R. L. (Mrs. A. D. McPherson)
Ross, M. I. (Mrs. J. L. Stewart)
Sampson, M. (Mrs. F. R. Archibald)
Seveigny, E. E. (Mrs. H. Lindley)
Shaw, M. A. (Mrs. Edward Nash)
Slee, V. E. (Mrs. J. Brown)
Snow, P. W. (Mrs. T. C. Read)
Stiles, M. K. (Mrs. Stewart Truman)
Swyers, B.
Swyers, Pearl
Swyers, Freda (Mrs. John Bailey)
Tennant, A. I. (Mrs. B. S. Johnston)
Wareham, J. B. (Mrs. T. Laurentius)
Walker, R. (Mrs. J. J. Brake)
Weldon, A. S. (Mrs. F. H. Goggin)
Wiechman, M. R. (Mrs. Roy Brown)
Willard, L. A. (Mrs. K. M. Goff)
Williams, D. I. (Mrs. D. Williams)

Class 1935

Angus, C. G.
Broadhurst, D. M. (deceased)
Brown, D. (Mrs. Ross Wright)
Burrow, M. (Mrs. E. Robbins)
Campderros, M.
Carter, O. R. (Mrs. G. Farrell)
Cowans, E.
Cunningham, J. (Mrs. Trevor Allison)
Fowler, E. T. (Mrs. B. A. W. Carter)
Greenwell, D. (Mrs. R. L. MacKinnon)
Grindley, E.
Hamilton, C. I. (Mrs. H. M. Dow)
Hanchet, F. (Mrs. F. H. Mitchell)
Howlett, M.
Israel, Lulu (Mrs. W. Kirk)
Kennedy, Joan (Mrs. J. Smith)
Lyford, L. V. (deceased)
Maclachlan, C. (Mrs. Philip Pascoe)
Michaels, A. (Mrs. C. H. Scharles) (deceased)
Mifflin, D. K. (Mrs. C. Penny)
Mimms, D. M. (Mrs. W. R. Gurling)
Morris, Muriel (Mrs. M. Hollett)
Moss, M.
Murphy, Ellen
Murphy, M. F. (Mrs. J. R. Levins)
Murray, R. W.
Ogilvie, M. D. (Mrs. C. Burns)
Parmenter, M. H. (Mrs. H. deBury)
Parsons, Fern (Mrs. R. Smith)
Pope, A. C.
Roberts, V. E. E. (Mrs. D. Filliter) (deceased)
Ross, C. G. (Mrs. Paterson-Smyth) (deceased)
Sandford, C. R. (Mrs. D. Findlay)
Scott, H. M. (Mrs. John McKeown)
Smith, W. K. (Mrs. H. R. Barker)
Thomson, L. M. (Mrs. L. A. Rounding)
Walker, P. E.
Welter, M. C. (Mrs. John Houston)
Whiteley, J.
Winsor, M. (Mrs. D. Cooper)
Worrall, B. I. (Mrs. R. R. Strong)
Young, E. A. (Mrs. E. Hoskins) (deceased)

Class 1936

Angel, H. C. (Mrs. G. Foley)
Bacon, P. E. R. (Mrs. G. Knapp)
Bjerketvedt, A. (Mrs. A. M. Webster)
Bunbury, M. K. (Mrs. W. H. Baker)
Case, J. L. (Mrs. F. W. Crowley)
Cole, H. E. (Mrs. J. H. Dundass)
Crockett, B. T.
Crombie, W. M. (Mrs. C. S. Adams)
Cullen, C. M. (Mrs. R. Clifford)
Chaplin, G. L. (Mrs. J. N. Houghton)
Darling, F. J. (Mrs. R. Ferguson)
Donnellan, M. I. (Mrs. Basil Eisenhaur)
Duchek, H. A. (Mrs. Leslie H. Wise)
Finnie, K. M. (Mrs. G. R. Brown) (deceased)
Fulton, M. I. (Mrs. Nick Berry)
Grant, M. K. (Mrs. Leonard Marcotte)
Haydon, M. B. (Mrs. M. Sutherland)
Higman, W. E. (Mrs. G. S. Ogilvie) (deceased)
Hill, M. E. (Mrs. T. S. Bennett)
Hodgson, E. A.
Hollett, C. R. (Mrs. R. Dancey)
Hudson, I. F.
Jamieson, D. A.
Jones, A. O. (Mrs. T. C. Brown)
King, C. C.
Lake, G. E. (Mrs. John E. Leishman)
LeBaron, E. R. (Mrs. George St. Pierre)
Montgomery, R. E.
Morrison, A. M.
Myers, R. M.
MacDonald, M. F.
MacKinnon, L. F. (Mrs. Norman Harris)
MacMillan, H. G. (Mrs. Fulton H. Copp)
McCormack, I. (Mrs. G. A. Kennedy)
McCutcheon, R. V.
McLeister, C. S.
McLeod, I. M.
McOuat, J. M. (Mrs. T. H. Wilkinson)
Niles, E. M. (Mrs. R. G. Shaw)
Pattillo, M. A. (Mrs. D. Roger)
Priestman, J. E. (Mrs. Sydney H. Holloway)
Sears, E. G. (Mrs. J. E. Gillespie)
Smith, J. M. (Mrs. Lewis Day)
Smith, M. H. (Mrs. E. D. Cooke)
Smith, P. E. E. (Mrs. B. A. Gamble)
Taylor, M. M. (Mrs. L. Ridgway)
Todd, M. I. (Mrs. H. Edgar)
Van Scoyoc, M. E.
Vaughan, V. I.
Watson, D. V.
Weston, E. M. E.

Class 1937

Adams, G. T.
Barton, E. G. (Mrs. J. R. Parkes)
Bayly, L. M. (Mrs. Howard Tewsley)
Betts, N. A. (Mrs. M. Silvester)
Blackler, M. J.
Brook, R. I. (Mrs. R. Seine)
Campbell, M. B. (Mrs. Berton Harper)
Carson, M. P.
Connor, P. M.
Cornish, E.
Cotton, D. B.
Cowan, N. D. (Mrs. Roger Mills)
Cox, P. (Mrs. Alex. Walker)
Elliott, J. W. (Mrs. Keith Horner)
Fife, L. M.
Fitzgerald, G. B.
Fritz, C. E.
Frost, D. G. (Mrs. Wayne Small)
Fuller, T. G. (Mrs. Harold H. Wallace)
Gray, J. L.
Hamilton, B. M. (Mrs. Stuart Bowes)
Hare, K. F. (Mrs. George Murphy)

APPENDIX C

Class 1937—Continued

Harvie, I. M. (Mrs. J. A. Johnston)
Hawley, E. P. (Mrs. Joseph Fiorito)
Hickman, H. T.
Jamieson, C. B. (Mrs. C. Knight)
King, M. A. (Mrs. M. A. Lyons)
Lane, M. I.
Marshall, C. (Mrs. M. Hoyt)
Martin, M. (Mrs. Austin Lush)
Miller, L. I.
Moulton, E. A. (Mrs. Raymond Churchey)
Murray, D. E. (Mrs. A. N. Inglis)
MacDonald, K. (Mrs. J. Wilson)
McLauchlan, A. B.
Pae, A. M.
Pasmore, H. L. (Mrs. W. R. Hart)
Paterson, M. G.
Pearle, S. M. (Mrs. P. Gitnick)
Post, A. I. (Mrs. G. Bjorkland)
Robinson, E. A. (Mrs. H. Russell)
Snider, I. L. (Mrs. J. MacDougall)
Sproule, R. E.
Talbot, M. L. (Mrs. John C. Newman)
Thurber, M. A. (Mrs. H. Althouse)
Tracey-Gould, M. E. (Mrs. J. E. Robinson)
Train, E. F. (Mrs. Joseph A. Head)
Tuttle, M. J.
Umphrey, V. R. (Mrs. H. Roy Bocock)
Vowles, M. R. (Mrs. Eric Millroy)
Wilson, D. E. (Mrs. L. Pearson)
Wright, E. S. (Mrs. W. Webster)
Young, C. M. J. (Mrs. C. Pullen)

Class 1938

Aikin, R. C.
Braithwaite, D. E. (Mrs. C. G. Motherwell)
(deceased)
Carmichael, T. J. (Mrs. C. F. M. Turfus)
Courtney, M. P. (Mrs. G. G. W. Lewis)
Dakin, D. I. (Mrs. Don Campbell)
Darby, B. R. (Mrs. C. R. Hawley)
Dayman, J. H.
Dixon, M. E. (Mrs. M. K. MacGougan)
Duthie, J. B. (Mrs. Carl Bischoff)
Eardley-Wilmot, B. R. (Mrs. G. Constable)
Fairweather, M. E. (Mrs. F. M. Bourne)
Fallon, R. M. (Mrs. J. Hill)
Farmer, M. M.
Farquhar, M. A. (Mrs. R. N. McCarthy)
Fee, P. M. (Mrs. J. B. St. Johns)
Flanagan, E. D. (Mrs. E. Jones)
Foreman, M. A. (Mrs. E. Turcot)
Gray, J. G. (Mrs. James F. Hughes)
Groom, M. M. (Mrs. H. R. Grout)
Harpell, M. K. (deceased)
Hayes, H. C.
Hennigar, S. F.
Hornibrook, M. A.
Jamieson, E. T. (Mrs. E. Amory)
Miller, F. E.
Milligan, V. (Mrs. H. S. Paul)
Morgan, O. G.
MacLatchey, F. M. (Mrs. H. R. Hudston)
MacPherson, M. E. (Mrs. Everett Dickson)
MacQuarrie, M. N. (Mrs. George deBelle)
McCann, M. J.
McElhanney, H. L. (Mrs. D. A. Thompson)
McLeod, M. K. (Mrs. Ian MacLennan)
McPhee, M. L. (Mrs. J. F. Fleming)
Neal, C. N. (Mrs. Wm. White)
Paxton, I. I. (Mrs. Keith Richan)
Reay, P. M.
Ross, J. C. (Mrs. J. MacDonald)
Savage, J. (Mrs. B. H. Moore)
Sawers, G. M. (Mrs. A. S. Veysey)
Scott, H. A. (Mrs. Claire Locke)
Sunderland, D. D. (Mrs. F. Birch)

Class 1938—Continued

Tennant, L. E. (Mrs. F. M. Dann)
Waller, M. G. (Mrs. Preston Robb)
Whitton, P. I. (Mrs. R. Fleet)
Willcocks, D. P. (Mrs. Chas. W. Kenick)
Woolmer, E. M. Z.

Class 1939

Allison, M. J. (Mrs. M. H. Bush)
Armour, E. B. (Mrs. Donald Lord)
Armstrong, S. B. (Mrs. S. Bean)
Ascah, D. L. (Mrs. D. Thomas)
Baird, B. C. (Mrs. Wm. Gibson)
Bamford, B. M. (Mrs. Duncan Chatfield)
Bates, V. O.
Betts, M. S.
Bishop, E. D.
Bray, M. E. (Mrs. Douglas Hutton)
Brotherston, K. A.
Brown, M. T. (Mrs. M. Pallister)
Campbell, F. J. (Mrs. C. O. Stinson)
Christian, H. E.
Clarke, M. H. (Mrs. Bruce A. T. Henry)
Clifford, K. H.
Cloran, M. F. E. (Mrs. Bain Currie)
Cluff, L. M. (Mrs. Roy C. McGee)
Clunie, M. E. F. (Mrs. E. Jamieson)
Corbett, M. H. (Mrs. W. Danik)
Craig, A. B. (Mrs. R. B. Harvey)
Dick, T. A. (Mrs. A. Stone)
Doherty, C. E.
Fawthrop, J. A. (Mrs. J. Marcelles)
Fee, A. L. (Mrs. R. Mills)
Fleming, A. S. (Mrs. J. Deming)
Freeze, M. E. A. (Mrs. A. Noble)
Froats, H. E. (Mrs. D. E. McClellan)
Gaskin, M. E. (Mrs. W. D. Stewart)
Greenlaw, D. I. (Mrs. D. Smith)
Halliday, M. V. (Mrs. M. Chase)
Hebb, P. J. (Mrs. J. Dickle)
Hebert, H. I. (Mrs. R. LaRoche)
Henderson, R. L. (Mrs. R. Charleson)
Hiltz, G. L. (Mrs. G. Meiklejohn)
Jacobs, D. S. (Mrs. G. R. Hornig)
Lindsay, M. E. (Mrs. Donald Ross)
Lutes, I. M. (Mrs. W. H. Oliver)
Little, E. C. (Mrs. John A. Tait)
deMerrall, P. C. (Mrs. W. H. Philip Hill)
Miles, D. M. (Mrs. D. Henschell)
Moore, F. B. (Mrs. Gerald Gale)
Motherwell, I. (Mrs. W. H. Lohnes)
MacDonald, M. M. (Mrs. Edwin Vowles)
MacDougall, G. A.
McGillis, M. H. (Mrs. J. J. Hatley)
MacLaren, A. I. (Mrs. K. Clarke)
MacLean, M. S. (Mrs. N. C. Root)
MacMillan, J. (Mrs. H. Edgar Morrison)
MacRae, J. K. (Mrs. J. Medine)
McElroy, T. P. (Mrs. Wylie T. Sharp)
Partington, C. A.
Pibus, O. M. (Mrs. R. Rice)
Picken, J. M. (Mrs. A. L. Danforth)
Randell, F. A. (Mrs. E. Brophy)
Reid, E. N.
Roberton, J. M. (Mrs. J. Dunfield)
Ross, E. F. (Mrs. A. J. Foote)
Runnells, M. J. (Mrs. B. H. Hill)
Schayltz, J. R. (Mrs. A. M. Forster)
Schroeder, E. C.
Scott, J. V. (Mrs. D. H. Mount)
Scott, M. E. (Mrs. James A. Dunlap)
Scott, Ruth, (Mrs. David R. Patchell)
Seeley, M. J. (Mrs. G. Tremblay)
Trump, Joan (Mrs. J. Playfair)
Willett, M. (Mrs. D. Ian Angus)
Wilton, H. M. (Mrs. John MacMillen)
Woodburn, G. L. L. (Mrs. J. W. Swift)

133

Class 1940

Andrews, Julia J. (Mrs. J. Milligan)
Armstrong, Catherine I. V. (deceased)
Atkinson, Dorothea R.
Barclay, Dorothy R.
Broadhurst, Barbara A. (Mrs. S. J. Porter)
Browne, Margaret A. (Mrs. D. Sutherland)
    (deceased)
Chalmers, Jessie M. (Mrs. J. B. Sheridan)
Christie, Anna A.
Clarkson, Louise C. (Mrs. Herbert D. Mintun)
Cleland, Allison C. (Mrs. Harry Minard)
Coulter, Phyllis M. (Mrs. W. Rothwell)
Daly, Elizabeth R. (Mrs. D. E. Haynes)
Dolan, Eunice O. (Mrs. J. McCaffrey)
Doull, Alix E. I.
Earle, Mary B. (Mrs. Donald Dunlop)
Ellis, Audrey A. (Mrs. C. W. Stanley)
Farmer, Louise F. (Mrs. E. Decker)
Findlay, Constance B. (Mrs. Harold Laxson)
Finnie, Alice B. (Mrs. Ross Walker)
Francis, Ruth C.
Gilker, Mary M. (deceased)
Harkness, Mary C. (Mrs. Maurice Elder)
Hebb, Katherine L. (Mrs. Gerald Halpenny)
Hill, Katherine S.
Hollett, Ella M.
Kindle, Katharine H. (Mrs. Douglas Smith)
Kinnear, Beatrice W. (Mrs. Bertie Burgess)
Labrèque, Esmé S.
Lindsay, Grace A. (Mrs. Charles F. Hyndman)
Little, Hilaire
Lovett, Phyllis F. (Mrs. P. Wilson)
Martinello, Adelene J. (Mrs. Charles E. Pressley)
Miller, Florence M. (Mrs. W. R. Mason)
Montgomery, Olive C. (Mrs. W. M. Wickland)
Murray, Catherine S.
MacDonald, F. Janet (Mrs. R. B. MacKenzie)
MacDonald, Flora W. (Mrs. H. R. Giberson)
MacDonald, Irene (Mrs. Harold MacDonald)
MacLeod, Alice W. (Mrs. Alice Dubuc)
MacQuarrie, Mary O. (Mrs. Charles Begg)
McCrindle, Gladys H. (Mrs. S. Sawry)
McEwen, Emma (Mrs. Robert Robertson)
McNair, Jean (Mrs. Norman Brown)
McOuat, Edith W. (Mrs. James Knox)
Patterson, Phyllis A. M. (Mrs. R. MacMorine)
Reid, Doretta J. (Mrs. J. Smart)
Scott, Ann M. J. (Mrs. Fred Jennings)
Seivewright, Agnes
Sherlock, Eileen E. (deceased)
Simms, Edith M. (Mrs. Donald Kimball)
Smallman, Marion E. (Mrs. Bruce Scriver)
Stuart, Jean C. (Mrs. M. Chandler)
Trueman, Margaret H.
Walker, Mary E. O. (Mrs. A. A. McCloy)
Wallace, Haroldene M. (Mrs. James Brown)
Williams-Guy, E. A. Lillian (Mrs. L. Bartlett)
Wheeler, Margaret M.
Worrall, Doris G. (Mrs. Randolph House)

Class 1941

Abbott, M. A. (Mrs. E. A. Dobson)
Acton, L. E. (Mrs. J. MacDonald)
Adam, B. M. (Mrs. S. Arnold) (deceased)
Anderson, M. J.
Beaugrand, E. B. (Mrs. Hugh St. Laurent)
Bennett, M. W. (Mrs. L. H. Marshall)
Briard, A. K. (Mrs. D. Smith)
Brown, A. D. (Mrs. H. B. Stoker)
Burgess, D. M. (Mrs. J. T. Fountain)
Caldwell, R. M. (Mrs. Clarence Stark)
Callanan, L. F. (Mrs. John Heenan)
Cavers, E. L. (Mrs. E. L. O'Kelly) (deceased)
Darling, B. E. (Mrs. B. E. Owen)

Class 1941—Continued

Eagleson, E. M. (Mrs. N. B. Delbel)
Ellard, L. J. (Mrs. T. A. D. Haddow)
Fraser, F. A.
Fraser, I. C. (Mrs. John Cunningham)
Gardner, K. E. (Mrs. Charles Smythies)
Graham, C. M. (Mrs. M. Durant)
Harper, M. M. (Mrs. M. M. Bragge)
Harris, R. E.
Harrison, E. M. (Mrs. W. S. Simpson)
Hawke, J. E. (Mrs. John Halliday)
Ings, L. M. (Mrs. B. Blodgett)
Jacobs, J. C.
Kelly, M. M. (Mrs. Frank Ker)
Knecht, J. B. (Mrs. R. L. Williams)
Kobayashi, M. C. (Mrs. M. Hecht)
Laite, A. B. A. (Mrs. E. Churchill)
Larmour, G. A. (Mrs. A. E. Crockett)
Lawton, J. M. (Mrs. M. L. Byers)
Linklater, A. G. (Mrs. Wm. Fry)
MacKenzie, M. C. (deceased)
Mahoney, M. G. (Mrs. A. P. Owens)
Mayville, M. V. (Mrs. J. E. Murphy)
MacDonald, M. E. (Mrs. John Ray Stobo)
MacLatchey, G. P. (Mrs. Reay M. Black)
MacLennan, M. A. (Mrs. M. A. Connor)
McCausland, I. P. (Mrs. P. Fitzgerald)
MacRae, I. F. (Mrs. H. T. Williams)
McDonald, M. J. (Mrs. Daniel Walsh)
Perram, M. V. (Mrs. I. Johnston)
Price, E. A.
Ruddock, C. E. (Mrs. Lloyd Thomas)
Sanderson, M. J. (Mrs. Kenneth Shaver)
Scott, E. M. (Mrs. Owen Bowland)
Starkey, E. E. (Mrs. W. H. Newel)
Tannahill, E. E. (Mrs. E. J. Richey)
Tupper, M. M.
Weir, M. C. (Mrs. M. MacDonald)
Weston, C. B. (Mrs. Claude Searcy)
Weston, M. B. (Mrs. C. H. B. Johnson)
Williams, E.
Wiseman, H. A. (Mrs. P. W. Holloway)
Zinck, M. M. (Mrs. Ralph Tracy)

Class 1942

Beaton, Mrs. Lydia (Mrs. D. Boyd)
Beek, Marcia (deceased)
Blackstock, A. Ruth (Mrs. Kenneth Narsted)
Brogan, Mildred M.
Buffett, Florence E. (Mrs. Milton Parsons)
Clarke, Mary (Mrs. Ian MacDonald)
Cox, Kathleen (Mrs. George Mills)
Crouse, Vivian L.
Derby, Kathleen E. (Mrs. Kenneth Carruthers)
Dixon, E. Vivian (Mrs. D. Bocking)
Dorning, Jean M. (Mrs. J. Sampson)
Fairweather, Nancy P. (Mrs. T. Wiggins)
Fraser, Allison P. (Mrs. L. W. Goodwin)
Fraser, Janet (Mrs. John Fox)
Gibson, Isobel D. (Mrs. J. R. Caverhill)
Goodwin, Elizabeth E. (Mrs. Kenneth Taylor)
Hall, M. Jean
Harrison, Margaret (Mrs. J. T. Robertson)
Hayward, Kathleen N. (Mrs. Hal Ritchie)
Hibbard, Elfrida I. (Mrs. William Payson)
Hillman, Elsie (Mrs. Douglas Thompson)
Ingram, Eileen
Innes, Audrey H. (Mrs. W. W. Wilson)
Johnson, Doreen B. (Mrs. J. Dodge)
Johnston, Isobel E. (Mrs. J. E. Macintyre)
Knowlton, Alida O. (Mrs. James W. Farrell)
Kydd, Elizabeth B. (Mrs. L. Sharp)
Laughlin, M. S. (Mrs. T. S. Tibo)
LeBrooy, Adorie W. (Mrs. A. Waygood)
Lefebvre, Corrine M. (Mrs. C. W. Depow)
Legere, B. M. (Mrs. R. P. MacKenzie)

Class 1942—Continued

Miller, Katherine H. (Mrs. C. E. H. Franklin)
Molson, Janet B. (Mrs. J. B. Sullivan)
Moore, Edythe L. (Mrs. J. D. McIntosh)
Morrison, Mary E. (Mrs. W. T. Thomas)
McCullough, Thirza T. (Mrs. John A. McCormick)
McLeod, H. B. (Mrs. John W. McMartin)
Neill, Rosamond W.
O'Regan, Mary L. (Mrs. Daniel Muir)
Parsons, Jean L. (Mrs. Rupert Doehler)
Pavlaskova, Marie
Perkins, E. Glenrose (Mrs. S. Blake Duffett)
Pugh, Julia G. (Mrs. W. R. Harvey)
Quenville, Rita M.
Saxton, Mildred E. (deceased)
Schroeder, Elsie H. (Mrs. E. Blackburn)
Schryer, Marjorie D. (Mrs. A. J. Francis)
Smeltzer, Miriam B. (Mrs. J. P. Chumbly)
Smith, Florence M. (Mrs. Reed H. Barnes)
Stanton, Nora A. (Mrs. Walter Blandy)
Stewart, Olive L.
Sweezey, Frances H. (Mrs. H. S. Henemander)
Thomas, Barbara J.
Thomas, Phyllis E.
Todd, Margaret E.
Van Bommel, Molly (Mrs. L. G. Easterbrook)
Wallace, Margaret (Mrs. Claude A. Mallett)
Wilbur, Luella R. (Mrs. Geo. A. Robinson)
Wilson, R. M. (Mrs. E. H. Sangwine)

Class 1943

Allen, F. M.
Baptist, L. H.
Bell, J. I. (Mrs. Bruce Currie)
Bishop, P. I. (Mrs. Ronald Meyer)
Black, B. E. (Mrs. A. C. Lambe)
Blais, J. R.
Brown, E. A. (Mrs. R. J. Kimmerly)
Browne, J. E. (Mrs. A. Fulton)
Burt, M. D. (Mrs. A. L. Leinback)
Cameron, L. K. (Mrs. R. M. Lane)
Cameron, P. C. (Mrs. Joseph Morley)
Canning, J. R. (Mrs. G. Robinson)
Chalmers, M. H. (Mrs. M. S. Milne)
Chornobrywy, E. M. (Mrs. C. Karpluk)
Clarkson, J. D. (Mrs. B. G. Miller)
Colley, E. H.
Connor, A. B. (Mrs. G. Gianfranceschi)
Dow, H. L. (Mrs. Robert Collier)
Fleming, M. A. (Mrs. James Westbecker)
Franklin, D. B.
Gardner, M. F. (Mrs. N. R. Hutt)
Gayler, E. M.
Gillis, L. M. (Mrs. C. Galbraith)
Gray, E. J. (Mrs. A. McM. Thompson)
Groundwater, E. F. (Mrs. A. J. Langley)
Hammond, E. P. (Mrs. John F. Haggerty)
Hicks, D. M. (Mrs. S. F. Curry)
Hunter, A. E. (Mrs. T. Porter)
Hunter, D. J. (Mrs. W. S. Weaver)
Kimpton, D. K. (Mrs. Ernest Bakewell)
Knoll, M. J.
Maile, V. M. (Mrs. Tony Falling)
Mersereau, L. E.
Moore, D. F. (Mrs. Raymond Haslam)
Morrison, D. J. (Mrs. J. Reilly)
Munro, E. E.
MacGillivary, A. C. (Mrs. Gordon MacDonald)
MacLeod, M. E. (Mrs. W. Menzies)
MacLeod, M. Miriam (Mrs. W. S. Livingstone)
MacNearney, J. E. (Mrs. J. Wallace)
MacCready, E. G.
McDermott, M. S. (Mrs. H. E. McCullough)
McNaughton, K. M. (Mrs. Norman Cumming)
McPhail, J. T.
Odell, F.

Class 1943—Continued

Pearson, M. M. (Mrs. R. G. Buckingham)
Pope, N. M. (Mrs. W. G. Carson)
Randall, D. E. (Mrs. Alex. Glen-Esh)
Read, M. L. (Mrs. Scott Miller)
Rideout, A. F. (Mrs. David M. Cook)
Shaw, E. P. (Mrs. K. Carton)
Sifton, M. R. (Mrs. E. MacCallum)
Snider, M. C. (Mrs. J. Sandilands)
Spence, W. C. (Mrs. Robert Stateson)
Stewart, D. P. (Mrs. James Bell)
Thompson, H. E. (Mrs. B. H. Utley)
Turner, B. A. (Mrs. C. McLachlan)
Walker, K. A.
Wallace, G. A. (Mrs. Walter Leggat)
Ward, Mary (Mrs. A. D. Morgan)
Watson, M. L. (Mrs. C. F. Lagasse)
Weeks, D. H. (Mrs. D. MacDowell)
Williams, G. E. (Mrs. J. Trainor)

Class 1944

Andrews, Verna L. (Mrs. E. R. E. Carter)
Annett, Elizabeth M. (Mrs. Edward Waddell)
Berens, Lyn R. (Mrs. D. Cash)
Bolton, Margaret (Mrs. Wm. Goodall)
Bowler, Margaret J. (Mrs. M. Robertson)
Cameron, Carolyn V. (Mrs. Myles Plecash)
Carr, Madeleine I. (Mrs. W. E. Stinson)
Curran, Margaret U. (Mrs. Vincent Delaney)
Curran, Marcella A.
Chute, Marion Edith (Mrs. B. A. H. Cartwright)
Davis, Eleanor F. (Mrs. Harold Williams)
Davis, Gertrude F. (Mrs. Roy Jack)
Ford, Marie Janet (Mrs. K. Luttrell)
Geldert, Roberta Louise (Mrs. F. Powers)
Grant, Shirley Hope (Mrs. Peter Freer)
Hawley, Beryle (Mrs. Raymond Moore)
Hamilton, Vivian M.
Hollingworth, Florence May
Hood, Eleanor C. (Mrs. D. G. McMillan)
Irven, Agnes (Mrs. A. Sawyer)
Jackson, Muriel Alice (Mrs. Stuart Berry)
Kitchen, Rowena P.
Larmour, E. Eleanore (Mrs. Charles Illick)
Moore, Margaret A. (Mrs. J. A. Blades)
MacDonald, Anna Ruth (Mrs. Francis Blake)
MacDonald, Jean (Mrs. M. C. Arnold)
MacDougall, Jonete (Mrs. Thomas Bailey)
McRae, Mary C.
McTavish, Myrtle (Mrs. Jack Forbes)
Newton, Mary Louise (Mrs. E. H. Knatchbull-Hugessen)
Royle, Beatrice M. (Mrs. John Gaw)
Roome, Barbara G.
Seybold, Mary Margery (Mrs. George Parker)
Simonson, Agnes L. (Mrs. C. E. Henry)
Skeete, Audrey R. (Mrs. A. Thomas)
Steele, Elspeth S. (Mrs. M. Putnam)
Surgenor, Dorothy Mary
Templeman, Dorothy A.
Trecarten, Mildred E. (Mrs. Stewart Groves)
Verrall, Margaret N. (Mrs. S. K. Telford)
Wayling, Doris Hazeldean
Wentzell, Lorna M. (Mrs. Harry Eisenhauer)
Woolward, Joy Muriel (Mrs. H. B. Humphreys)
Wright, Kathleen M. (deceased)
Whitehead, M. W. (married)

Class 1945

Ackers, Elizabeth F. (Mrs. E. Carter)
Aitkens, Elizabeth
Arkwright, Eileen G. (Mrs. D. N. McSween)
Barclay, Lillian H.
Barnhill, Eva F. (Mrs. Malcolm J. MacLean)

Class 1945—Continued

Baxter, Evelyn L. (Mrs. H. Hilton)
Bigelow, E. Welthea (Mrs. John Smardon)
Boon, Doris M. (Mrs. Patrick Holden)
Bowles, Beverly F. (Mrs. G. R. Lauer)
Caldwell, Dorothy E. (Mrs. D. McCallister)
Carr, Annie C. (Mrs. Warren W. Ingalls)
Chandler, Joan B. (Mrs. H. A. Wilson)
Corner, H. Maureen (Mrs. J. B. Stevens)
Dahms, Phyllis I. (Mrs. John Shepley)
Donaghy, June E. (Mrs. J. T. Gavriloff)
Everson, Margaret E. (Mrs. George Campbell)
Fawthrop, Annie K. (Mrs. R. Gibson)
Fitzgerald, Margaret M. (Mrs. D. Kenney)
Fraser, Dorothy M. (Mrs. L. R. Gould)
Fulton, Jean R. (Mrs. G. Rawluk)
Gardiner, Nanette (Mrs. J. W. Stannix)
Halsey, Peggy L. (Mrs. R. G. Green)
Hamilton, Ada M.
Hearle, Drucilla
Heatlie, Evelyn D. (Mrs. G. G. Garrioch)
Hillborg, Beaulah G. (Mrs. A. G. Bellaire)
Jardine, Virginia G. (Mrs. Harold Lockerbie)
Johnston, Mable N. (married)
Kingman, Mrs. Gwyneth G.
Levigne, Dorothy H. (Mrs. Bruce T. Gillespie)
Lisson, Elizabeth H. (Mrs. R. G. Corkran)
Lisson, Jean I. (Mrs. Edward Chaplin)
Loach, Virginia E. (Mrs. C. McCulley)
Mabee, Margaret
Merritt, Edith-Barbara (Mrs. G. Jamer)
Miles, Olive B. (Mrs. Bruce Giles)
Morrow, Joan I. (Mrs. S. Langille)
Morrow, Margaret S.
Motherwell, Hilda C. (Mrs. N. F. Bradley)
Muff, Janet (Mrs. George Stunden)
Munro, Lillian B.
MacDonald, Doris I. (Mrs. Harold Gunter)
MacDonald, Edith C. (Mrs. E. Sperry)
MacDuff, Irene (Mrs. David High)
MacLennan, Janet (married)
McDougall, Audrey A. (Mrs. David Rennie)
McEwen, Alethea G. (Mrs. Karl Porter)
McLeod, Meriam I. (Mrs. Garth Mosher)
McLean, Vivian A. (Mrs. C. Nixon)
McKee, Norma E. (Mrs. Ernest Harnish)
Palmer, Joan (Mrs. G. Whittock)
Parsons, B. Gwendolyn (Mrs. Douglas Bet)
Price, Marjorie (Mrs. M. Tuttie)
Ramsey, Dorothea E. (Mrs. R. E. Jess)
Redpath, Marjorie N. (Mrs. T. Bridge)
Reilley, Margaret F. (Mrs. T. Mulligan)
Robson, Marjorie S. (Mrs. Wm. Hutchison)
Royston, Romayne M. (Mrs. Michael Mulvihill)
Shea, Ada F.
Skaftved, Elsie (Mrs. Wm. Burton)
Sly, Isobel C. (Mrs. J. H. Rooks)
Smith, Inez (Mrs. R. Leathwood)
Soles, Jean O. (Mrs. Arnold Elliott)
Tackaberry, Marjorie H. (Mrs. Ivan Montgomery)
Tainsh, Patricia (Mrs. P. Marino)
Todd, Thelma (Mrs. G. A. Legassic)
Walker, Aurelia (Mrs. A. Phillips-Woolley)
Watson, Elizabeth F.
Wilkinson, Dorothy M. (married)
Willett, Ruth A. (Mrs. James Long)
Wilson, Corinne A. (Mrs. C. A. Cameron)
Woodward, Margery H.
Yearsley, Margaret E. (Mrs. Wm. M. Johnston)

Class 1946

Alexander, Lorna J. (Mrs. Walter Hood)
Ames, Charlotte E. (deceased)
Ashbourne, Louise B. (Mrs. C. Howard Simpkin)
Atkinson, Kathleen M. (Mrs. Joseph Hendry)

Class 1946—Continued

Beaton, June M. (Mrs. Harold Lawton)
Bethel, Doreen M. (Mrs. R. Stanton)
Bjornlund, H. Elizabeth
Bradford, Shirley M. (Mrs. S. Hill)
Calnek, Beatrice C. (Mrs. Herbert McGee)
Cartmel, Priscilla H. (Mrs. M. Devlen)
Coates, Pauline M.
Conroy, Dorothy (Mrs. Jack Sadler)
Conroy, Hilda C. (Mrs. Wm. Wilson)
Coons, Madge E.
Cotton, E. Pauline
Critchley, Mary F. (Mrs. D. A. McVicar)
Dorning, Margaret R. (Mrs. P. Brayshaw)
Findlay, H. Marie (Mrs. Stewart MacKenzie)
Ford, H. Vera (Mrs. E. Gill)
Gagnon, Helen M. (Mrs. Jack Muir)
Goodall, Jean R. (Mrs. Jean Hanchet)
Gove, Stella R. (Mrs. F. E. Wherley)
Hopkins, Audrey E. (Mrs. A. Hopkins)
Hurren, Muriel C. (Mrs. Geo. Lorimer)
Jackson, Norma P. (Mrs. D. M. Bryant)
Jamieson, Elizabeth
Jepson, Evelyn G. (Mrs. Clyde Forbes)
Johnson, Sybil G. (Mrs. T. Fields)
Lonergan, Evelyn M. (Mrs. Peter Palmer)
Major, Agnes G. (Mrs. Wm. D. MacDonald)
Major, Elizabeth M. (Mrs. John Mole)
Marmon, Marguerite E. (Mrs. Gregor MacLeod)
Mason, Joan D. (Mrs. I. D. MacKenzie)
Miller, Jean (Mrs. Thomas Peake)
Moffatt, Doris E.
Morrison, Norma J. (Mrs. L. E. Copleston)
Morton, Euphemia C. (Mrs. E. Campbell)
MacIntosh, Joyce M. (Mrs. P. B. Savory)
MacLachlan, Joan B. (Mrs. Robert S. Green)
MacRae, Margaret J. (Mrs. J. Stewart Morton)
McGreer, Letitia M. (Mrs. John Snodgrass)
McIntosh, Catherine B. (Mrs. E. A. MacCallum)
McKimm, Barbara (Mrs. J. Beattie)
Nussey, Rosamond V.
O'Rourke, Doris E. (Mrs. G. R. Brine)
Philip, Muriel E. (Mrs. Irving C. Hall)
Pibus, Barbara M. (Mrs. E. A. S. Reid)
Pugh, Patricia M. (Mrs. Norman MacLean)
Robinson, Bessie G. (Mrs. Douglas Bell)
Rosser, Joan S. (Mrs. J. Roland)
Rowe, Nancy C. (Mrs. W. Dempster)
Salmon, Hazel
Sansom, L. Elizabeth (Mrs. E. L. Quirk)
Scott, Bernice E. (Mrs. Roger Miner)
Spearman, Eleanor G. (deceased)
Sproule, Winnifred (Mrs. M. H. Mudge)
Stevens, M. Jean (Mrs. B. Robertson)
Stewart, Phyllis K. (Mrs. Frank F. Smith)
Tomilson, Laura (Mrs. J. Y. Robichaud)
Tully, Anne J. (Mrs. C. F. Grant)
Van Vliet, G. Elizabeth (Mrs. P. R. Jones)
Virtue, Edythe T. (Mrs. D. C. Prowse)
Watters, Ann. I. (Mrs. R. Fillmore)
Webber, Edna (Mrs. Peter Barg)
Weston, Marguerite U. (Mrs. John Baker)
Wurtele, Mary T. (Mrs. M. Smith)
Yard, Helen A.

Class 1947

Aitken, Rahno A. (Mrs. Wm. Taylor)
Allan, Kathleen A. (Mrs. R. Playfair)
Armstrong, M. Eleanor (Mrs. A. Robertson)
Bailey, Isabelle D. (Mrs. Henry C. Adams)
Barberie, Muriel A. (Mrs. Muriel Peeler)
Beattie, Frances G. (Mrs. Porter Howard)
Beebe, Constance V. (Mrs. R. Rider)
Beginn, Doris L. (Mrs. Lewis Herberts)
Boulette, Ruth J. (Mrs. R. J. Birmingham)

Class 1947—Continued

Burroughs, Frances H. (Mrs. Ian Milne)
Byers, Joan (Mrs. R. J. Mullins)
Calnen, Florence S.
Campbell, Florence V. (Mrs. S. McParland)
Comber, Elaine M. (Mrs. E. M. Van Zanten)
Corey, Lucy A. (Mrs. G. Moore)
Corey, Phyllis E. (Mrs. Kenneth Haring)
Crouse, Pauline J. (Mrs. W. Naugler)
Danyluk, Anne (Mrs. R. Wachna)
Dickison, Evelyn M. (Mrs. Alan Bickford)
Driver, Helen S. (Mrs. Herbert Pragnell)
Earle, Elinore H. (Mrs. Burt B. Hale)
Eastwood, M. Joan (Mrs. Pierre Chevalier)
Forbes, F. Margaret
Fritch, Pauline M. (Mrs. Peter Schopflocher)
Ganten, Norma J. (married)
Gower-Rees, Mary
Gzowski, Edith
Hamilton, Shirley (Mrs. John Wm. Powers)
Helleur, Eileen B. (Mrs. Robert E. M. Hamilton)
Henchey, Barbara M. (Mrs. Edward Halischuk)
Hillborg, Norma L. (married)
Hines, Mary K. (married)
Hood, Ruth L. (Mrs. Louis Horlick)
Hooper, Helen L. (Mrs. H. W. D. Kilgour)
Howard, Laura D. (Mrs. Robert Oliver)
Jamieson, Sheila P. (Mrs. A. Dibblee)
Jensen, Iris C. M.
Kelly, Roberta E. (Mrs. Harry A. Shipman)
Kneeland, Marjorie J. (Mrs. David C. MacCallum)
Knowles, B. Joan (Mrs. J. R. Wright)
Knowles, Peggy P. (Mrs. Robert Perry)
Knox, Hylda D. (Mrs. George Dick)
Lamb, Helen T. (Mrs. John Shearman)
Leahy, Elizabeth E. (Mrs. E. Soderston)
Lewis, Margaret L.
Lynch, Theresa C.
MacKenzie, Audrey E.
MacKenzie, Florence I.
MacPherson, Jean S. (Mrs. R. St. John)
McClure, Helen M. (Mrs. R. S. Cameron)
McEwen, Ada E.
Moore, Gwendolyn G. (Mrs. Fred Reader)
Morrison, Elizabeth M. (Mrs. Preston McLean)
Myra, Ruth V. (Mrs. Robert C. Short)
Ramsey, Marguerite M. E. (Mrs. Ian M.
MacKinnon)
Reed, Jacqueline C. (Mrs. Robert Connors)
Rimmer, Margaret E. (Mrs. D. W. Edmunds)
Roy, Phyllis W. (Mrs. O. K. Lauren)
Sanderson, Celeste (Mrs. George Flight)
Smyth, Margaret M. (Mrs. Edward G. Mahon)
Stearns, Anne L. (Mrs. W. H. MacMillan)
Studd, Joan R. (Mrs. B. Koken)
Thorslund, Lillian E. (Mrs. R. G. Roche)
Todd, Betty L. (Mrs. Charles Walper)
Tomalty, Lorna G. (Mrs. B. Davis)
Tulk, Marie M. V. (Mrs. James B. Samson)
Walsh, Norah B. (Mrs. Allan W. Weir)
Walsh, R. Alison (Mrs. W. Alan Shaw)
Weisburgh, Hazel I. (Mrs. Norman H. Weiner)
Whalen, Joan M. (Mrs. L. J. Bilodeau)
Yearwood, June A.

Class 1948

Bell, Kathleen A. (Mrs. Wm. A. McGillivray)
Biard, Edna M. R. (Mrs. E. King)
Bingle, Joyce H. (Mrs. Charles Gibbons)
Bothwell, Jean D. (Mrs. Robert Tribe)
Boast, Lois M.
Bradley, Elizabeth (Mrs. P. A. Courage)
Blandford, Pauline A. (Mrs. Norman Derrick)
Brown, Gertrude E. (Mrs. G. B. Rutherford)
Chalmers, Elizabeth

Class 1948—Continued

Chisholm, Joan M.
Christian, Ethel E. (Mrs. Eric Bailey)
Craig, June (Mrs. J. Chang)
Dickinson, Helen C. (Mrs. G. K. Bennett)
Dixon, Muriel (Mrs. M. Spooner)
Ellis, Jean M. (Mrs. Robert Keep)
Firlotte, Ila F. (Mrs. J. McRae)
Glass, Frances M. (Mrs. D. Horner)
Hacking, Jean (Mrs. D. A. Deans)
Haldane, Catherine M. (Mrs. Roy D. MacNeill)
Hall, Caroline M. (Mrs. John C. Stubbs)
Hall, Dorothy
Hamilton, Elizabeth (Mrs. E. Norris)
Hanna, Margaret L. (Mrs. C. G. Willis)
Hase, Geraldine V. (Mrs. G. Tardif)
Hewson, Florence (Mrs. D. R. Carr)
Hiscock, Mabel (Mrs. Rupert Bartlett)
Hodgson, Anne R. (Mrs. W. N. Townley)
Johnson, Janet R. (Mrs. Wm. S. Martin)
Johnson, Margaret J. (Mrs. Ralph Gray McGaw)
Kean, Daphne C. E.
Knecht, Anna R. (Mrs. Gerald Walker)
Lambert, Marguerite M. (Mrs. M. M. Greening)
Leahy, Colleen (Mrs. Edward Pete)
Lee, Elsie A. M. (Mrs. Elwood Dick)
Letts, June (Mrs. Roy McCormack)
Letts, Ruth (Mrs. Frank Hughes)
Logie, Ruth (Mrs. Thomas Taylor)
Lusk, Lois E. (Mrs. Brock Batten)
Maguire, Melicent V.
Marston, Alberta (Mrs. L. J. Firing)
Meyers, Ruth (Mrs. Charles Tessier)
Miller, Shirley (Mrs. A. Robbins)
McCuaig, Marion (Mrs. Donald MacDonald)
McDougall, Mary (Mrs. Frank I. Ritchie)
McKnight, Mary E.
MacKenzie, Julia (Mrs. Hamilton Fish)
McLennan, Diana E. (Mrs. E. S. Cleland)
MacVicar, Isabel (Mrs. R. Skinner)
Norman, Ileana (Mrs. W. Rons)
O'Connell, Natalie (Mrs. S. T. Smeeth)
Parker, Ruth
Patterson, Josephine (Mrs. John Bermingham Jr.)
Patterson, Wanda E. (Mrs. Sydney Hay)
Penney, Dorothy S. (Mrs. D. Colter)
Pettingill, Wilma C. (Mrs. H. Van Nest Hoff)
Poole, Mary P. (Mrs. R. A. Biers)
Pritchard, Catherine (Mrs. A. McTavish)
Richardson, Anne E. (Mrs. J. H. Haldimand)
Riley, Irma K.
Rose, Norma P.
Shaw, Barbara J. (Mrs. Arthur Smialowski)
Shepherd, Marion M.
Smallshaw, Yvonne M. (Mrs. Ross Taylor)
Taylor, Adele F. (Mrs. J. Bell)
Taylor, Gaynor J. (Mrs. Raymond Ostlund)
Telford, Joan A. (Mrs. K. MacDonald)
Tomilson, Dallas E. (Mrs. Donald Morley)
Tomilson, Doris E. (Mrs. Frank Merrill)
Walker, Alice M. (Mrs. K. Home)
Watt, Evelyn E. (Mrs. E. E. Watt)
Welling, Shirley I. (Mrs. John Caron)
Wornell, Joan I. (Mrs. A. E. Norris)

Class 1949

Alexander, Patricia C.
Allen, Reta K. (Mrs. R. Martin)
Andersen, Eva
Bankart, Beverley (Mrs. Donald K. MacPhail)
Black, Elise K.
Brands, Barbara A. (Mrs. James W. Martin)
Brophy, Shirley M. (Mrs. Arthur G. Mackey)
Cameron, Betty E. (Mrs. A. E. Oliver)
Clarke, Beatrice (Mrs. B. Young)

137

Class 1949—Continued

Clarke, Vivian D. (Mrs. D. D. McIntosh)
Crook, Irma M. (Mrs. I. M. Jacobs)
Cummings, Elizabeth
Denman, Patricia M. (Mrs. Ronald A. Smith)
Dingwall, E. Jean (Mrs. Ian W. Gregory)
Donovan, M. Patricia (Mrs. J. H. A. Lawrence)
Dunn, Betty Marie
Filliol, Monique (Mrs. M. Macbeth)
Fisher, Lorna M. (Mrs. Robert MacLean)
Fisher, Marjorie (Mrs. Gordon Sutton)
Foster, Jean M. (Mrs. R. B. MacDonald)
Gage, Marion (Mrs. Howard W. Brummitt)
Graham, Catherine
Gray, Beverley (Mrs. Hugh Smith)
Harvey, Kathleen L.
Hayman, Patricia (Mrs. E. P. Moore)
Hume, Nancy J. (Mrs. Walter Bosse)
King, M. Joyce
Laughlin, Ruth (Mrs. Forbes McAslan)
McCune, Phyllis M. (Mrs. Richard P. Hipkin)
MacDonald, Bertha P. (Mrs. Ernest Grant)
McGregor, Margaret G. (Mrs. Vivian Villet)
MacKay, E. Joyce (Mrs. MacNaughton
                             Cummings)
MacKay, M. Jeannette (Mrs. Barry LePatourell)
MacLean, Ruth H.
MacLennan, Gladys E.
MacLeod, Dorothy K. (Mrs. D. K. Bracken)
MacWilliams, Joyce I. (Mrs. J. Bush)
Malcolm, Emily M. (Mrs. Lloyd Mitchell)
Mitchell, Harrietta
Monteith, Virginia E.
Morrison, Flora (Mrs. W. Archibald)
Munro, Mary (Mrs. David Miller)
Neeld, Ruth A. (Mrs. Kenneth C. Eaton)
Rankin, Barbara K.
Read, Muriel E.
Royle, Edith A. (Mrs. Allan Molyneaux)
Saint, Mary G. (Mrs. Charles Smith)
Scott, Margaret (Mrs. P. D. Bateman)
Seifert, Mildred (Mrs. M. Whaley)
Smith, Jean M. (Mrs. Bernard Lacroix)
Smith, Marjorie C.
Snetsinger, Anne R. (Mrs. Stuart H. Cool)
Stephen, Joyce M. (Mrs. Earl Bamford)
Thurston, Patricia (Mrs. Ross Bannerman)
Topp, Patricia (Mrs. Robert Orr)
Uhl, Betty L. (Mrs. George Woods)
Watling, Jean (Mrs. George Bradwell)
Woods, Dorothy A. (Mrs. Frank Brophy)
Wrigley, M. Joan
Wyman, Eleanor J. (Mrs. Robert Cook)

Class 1950

Arkwright, Beryl
Badgley, Elizabeth (Mrs. G. Graham)
Blandford, Margaret
Bosse, Lorraine
Britch, Norma Nokes
Clapham, Joan (Mrs. Daniel B. Harris)
Collis, Jacqueline A.
Connor, Claire E. (Mrs. J. R. Martin)
Cornelius, Ann (Mrs. John D. Woodward)
Davis, Norma L.
Day, Alice Mary (Mrs. Winfred Glass)
Deans, June E. (Mrs. W. Armstrong)
Deslauriers, Patricia E. (Mrs. Herbert Ott)
Duchesnay, Madeleine
Elder, Margaret D. (Mrs. George Flack)
Flett, Evelyn A.
Fuller, Anne F. (Mrs. W. Grauwiler)
Gerrish, Ann V. (Mrs. J. LaRue Wiley)
Gorssline, Ruth M. (Mrs. F. B. Cameron)
Hartland, Phyllis M.
Harvey, Audrey F. (Mrs. R. Koch)
Hebert, Helen E.

Class 1950—Continued

Howard, Rona Elva (Mrs. Len Miller)
Johnston, Elizabeth (Mrs. Philip A. Wood)
Jones, Margaret G.
Keith, Joan C. (Mrs. George A. Goodwin)
Kerr, Marjorie B.
Loach, Grace (Mrs. Jack C. Sawyer)
Lennon, Dorothy E.
Miller, Catherine (Mrs. V. McCreight)
Moore, Catherine H. (Mrs. John MacGregor)
Morris, Pamela J. (Mrs. J. E. Leach)
Morton, Shirley E.
MacDonald, Myrtle M. (Mrs. Willard Greene)
McFarland, Verna M. (Mrs. A. Crittenden)
McGibbon, Barbara H.
MacLeod, Bernice (Mrs. James T. Fall)
McMillan, Christina R.
Palmer, Margaret L. (Mrs. M. L. Estabrooks)
Parker, Doreen
Perkins, Janet T. (Mrs. S. Rutherford)
Pike, Flora I.
Prescott, Anne F. (Mrs. Wm. Cooke)
Ritcey, Barbara A. (Mrs. Frank Staskow)
Robertson, Diane A. (Mrs. Arthur Walter)
Robertson, Ruby D. M.
Rowan, Jean C.
Russell, Sheila M. (Mrs. R. McKenna)
Scott, Willa Jane (Mrs. Jack Temple)
Skutezky, Eva M.
Sly, Evelyn J.
Smith, Jeanne F. (Mrs. Ralph Matthews)
Steele, Jean C. (Mrs. Russell Anderson)
Talbot, Evelyn Lois (Mrs. R. Laselle)
Tarrant, Mae-Louise (Mrs. K. A. McPhatter)
Tilton, Barbara G.
Wilcox, Mary Elizabeth (Mrs. Nelson Allatt)
Woodruff, June W. (Mrs. S. H. Woodend)
Worrall, Doris Irene (Mrs. Jack Bromilow)
Wulffraat, J. Margaret (Mrs. R. H. McColl)
Wyman, Elmina C. (Mrs. A. Kemp)

Class 1951

Agnes, Doris H. (Mrs. Leonard De Wolfe)
Ascah, Elizabeth (Mrs. S. B. Jones)
Banas, Wanda (Mrs. Wilson Drew)
Bennett, Lois M. (Mrs. L. Carriere)
Berry, Gwendolyn M. (Mrs. Alan J. Greer)
Bingley, Joan E. (Mrs. John A. McGillis)
Bodnaruk, Julia (Mrs. Albert Mensour)
Bryson, Mary I. (Mrs. Kenneth Younie)
Burgoyne, Mary
Cassidy, Margaret (Mrs. M. Prizant)
Chapman, Freda (Mrs. F. Leonard)
Charlton, Audrey (Mrs. Alastair Cameron)
Cooke, Beverley (Mrs. Roy Juneau)
Cooper, Dorothy E. (Mrs. Bruce McCullogh)
Curtis, Effie M. (Mrs. T. B. Philips)
Davidson, Joan M. (Mrs. Robert Marshall)
Deacon, Isabel L. (Mrs. Robert H. Grasby)
Erskine, Grace E. (Mrs. Sterling J. McLeod)
Ferguson, Patricia E. (Mrs. N. W. Joyce)
Forin, Lona A. (Mrs. Donald K. Clogg)
Freeborough, Anne (Mrs. Richard Price)
Gair, Joyce (Mrs. Charles M. Allan)
Gaudet, Jeannine L. (Mrs. James Adams)
Gerth, Shirley E.
Glass, Edna M. (Mrs. Wm. H. Lalonde)
Hamilton, Lorraine (Mrs. Jack Whiteley)
Harper, Helen J. (Mrs. D. A. Townsend)
Harrison, Pamela M. (Mrs. John Gaskill)
Helleur, Dorothy V. (Mrs. Oakley Bush)
Johnson, Anne S.
Jowsey, June B. (Mrs. Robert Bowley)
Kinnie, Shirley
Knapp, Anita J. (Mrs. David Boys)
Knight, Beatrice R.

Class 1951—Continued

Link, Barbara J. (Mrs. Jacques St. Amour)
Lucas, Elizabeth J. (Mrs. D. H. Stewart)
Lyons, Isabel (Mrs. Edward P. Walter)
McCoubrey, Joyce I. (Mrs. Ernest Penrose)
McDonald, Phyllis
MacKenzie, Elizabeth L. (Mrs. Wm. C. Forsyth)
McKinven, Roberta (Mrs. Philip C. Gale)
MacNaughton, Elizabeth (Mrs. E. Fox)
McWilliam, Anne E. (Mrs. M. S. Ladd)
Milligan, Merle
Mitchell, Margaret (Mrs. Frank King)
Mooney, Elizabeth J. (Mrs. R. A. Stevenson)
Moore, Patricia E. (Mrs. R. K. McCormack)
Morrison, Katherine M. (Mrs. Fred Frazer)
O'Neill, Rose T. (Mrs. R. T. Stacey)
Parkinson, Anne E. (Mrs. Wm. A. Clark)
Patterson, Patricia E. (Mrs. Leo Brocket)
Preston, Charlotte
Powles, Isabel C. (Mrs. J. G. Rowe)
Sangster, Georgena M. (Mrs. V. C. Havelock)
Schwartz, Helen S. (Mrs. Charles Pease)
Scott, Avery (Mrs. Ray Stanyar)
Slack, Helen (Mrs. M. A. Loiscone)
Stowe, Anita G. (Mrs. Neil H. Tattrie)
Stubbs, Evelyn (Mrs. R. C. Malcolm)
Vibert, Wilma S. (Mrs. H. F. Biehl)
Watt, Edith Grace
Wilbur, Marguerite (Mrs. John Fingland)
Wilson, Marion (Mrs. James L. Saunders)
Wishart, Reta V.

Class 1952

Abelson, Marion I. (Mrs. Derek M. Sharpe)
Akerley, Helen Mae (Mrs. Walter C. Wallis)
Alexander, Phyllis I. (Mrs Ronald Stanford)
Allen, Margaret R. (Mrs. M. R. Begbie)
Anderson, Jane (Mrs. Leslie A. McNicol)
Anderson, May C. (Mrs. Ernest Wilson)
Ashbourne, Bessie M. B.
Bennett, Frances I.
Bill, Margery A. E.
Bishop, Shirley M. (Mrs. E. R. Epp)
Bowden, Barbara A. (Mrs. B. A. Ellis)
Breeze, Beverley F. (Mrs. B. E. Ducat)
Bunbury, Marjorie S.
Burbank, J. Pearl (Mrs. R. R. Pearson)
Burns, Norma F.
Cameron, I. June (Mrs. Donald Curtis)
Clements, Elizabeth K. (Mrs. D. Grimes)
Clinton, Flora E. (Mrs. F. Ferguson)
Colquhoun, Louise M. (Mrs. Harry W. Webster)
Connors, Shirley M. (Mrs. Anthony A. Malo)
Corrigan, Joan H.
Crimp, Shirley E. (Mrs. Wm. J. Roberts)
Crue, Leitha R. (Mrs. Carl Thorston)
Dodge, Anna I. (Mrs. A. Vanier)
Donaldson, Margaret J.
Duhan, Mary K. (Mrs. Mary Elcox)
Dunn, Ivy
Gannon, Patricia M. (Mrs. Chas M. Hamilton)
Gillies, Anne D.
Greer, Dorothy J. (Mrs. D. Flitton)
Guest, Kaireen F. (Mrs. K. F. Allen)
Hamilton, Mary K.
Hodgson, Anne C. (Mrs. John W. Dennis)
Jolley, Yvonne
Laberee, Eleanor I. (Mrs. Lloyd A. Robertson)
Ladd, Audrey G.
Legge, Carroll
Lepine, M. Florence
Lovett, Lois H. (Mrs. Robert Laberge)
MacDonald, A. Catherine
MacDonald, Glenna I. (Mrs. David Calder)
MacKean, Josephine H. (Mrs. Alistair Gray)
MacKinnon, Grace M. (Mrs. Robert Hone)

Class 1952—Continued

MacLennon, Audrey C. (Mrs. A. C. Dostie)
MacNeil, Joan M. (Mrs. Joseph A. Aitkens)
Mills, Elizabeth B. (Mrs. A. E. Sesselberg)
Mooers, Maxime A.
Neville, Dallas L.
Overstrom, Barbro E.
Reed, Joan R. (Mrs. Sterling Harris)
Robinson, Joan M.
Rowat, Jean A. (Mrs. Kenneth Birch)
Rowland, Joan I. (Mrs. K. J. Thorneycroft)
Sanderson, Helen Ethel (Mrs. Robert Cooch)
Sims, Evelyn E. (Mrs. Torald Lutwick)
Smith, Norma W. (Mrs. Gerald Trineer)
Stairs, Dorothy H.
Tracy-Gould, Zora N. C. (Mrs. Zora Keddie)
Turner, Jessie (Mrs. John Dale Weldon)
Tyler, Anne R. (Mrs. Michael Hailing)
Woodward, Beverley A. (Mrs. Robert H. Strange)
Zinck, Barbara G.

Class 1953

Acton, Barbara E. (Mrs. L. W. Hersey)
Aitchison, Joan (Mrs. Sterling Mair)
Anjo, Norma (Mrs. Lennox Parr)
Barr, Norma M. (Mrs. C. M. Palmer)
Beckingham, Ann C.
Berry, Jean (Mrs. John Bufton)
Besidowski, Sophie (Mrs.
Bryan, Audrey L.
Bunce, Mary C. (Mrs. M. C. Beecroft)
Bush, Elizabeth A. (Mrs. B. A. MacDougall)
Butterworth, Joan E. (Mrs. James Ellemo)
Christie, Isabell
Colquhoun, Joan M. (Mrs. Roland Bodie)
Connery, Barbara (Mrs. Ralph Thriepland)
Donald, Ruth F. (Dr. Ruth Pankhurst)
Fitzgerald, Molly C. (Mrs. Paul Pritchard)
Forsyth, Elizabeth (Mrs. Randolph Burton)
Fullerton, Barbara (Mrs. John M. Gilmour)
Golden, Elizabeth B. (married)
Greer, Noreen (Mrs. Gordon C. Peters)
Haberl, Mary E. (Mrs. Charles A. Park)
Hargrove, Joanne P. (Mrs. Ronald Reeves)
Hersey, Elizabeth (Mrs. Byron Crozier)
Holmes, Norma (Mrs. Lorne Cox)
Jamieson, Shirley (Mrs. Hugh Montgomery)
King, Jean P. (Mrs. Fred Collins)
Kirkpatrick, Doris (Mrs. Harold Stymest)
Lavallee, Constance (Mrs. Frank R. Smith)
Lederer, Susanne F. (married)
LeMarquand, Sheryl E. (Mrs. Wm. John Kitson)
McCarthy, Sheila (Mrs. Michael Luciuk)
MacMillan, Norma
Major, Frances (Mrs. Eldon Dunning)
Mandigo, Dolores (Mrs. K. Baggott)
Mihelich, Albina (Mrs. Wallace Ellicott)
Mieszkowska, Jadwiga (Mrs. J. Szeliski)
Millward, Jean V.
Nakagawa, Chieko (Mrs. Paul Toyonaga)
O'Rourke, Audrey E. (Mrs. Wm. Gossage)
Oughtred, Janet A. (Mrs. Robert MacKinnon)
Parris, Ruth (Mrs. D. K. Wedderspoon)
Peacock, Grace (Mrs. Isaac Tuplin)
Pye, Jane Ann (Mrs. Lawrence Bergeron)
Ralph, Betty (Mrs. John D Sharp)
Ramier, Mary E. (Mrs. Nigel Charlong)
Rau, Ethel B.
Ross, Betty (Mrs. Walter Scott)
Savage, Shirley (Mrs. David Simms)
Smith, Frances
Smith, Sheila (Mrs. W. H. Alexander)
Standish, Hazel (deceased)
Stucker, Elizabeth
Taylor, Helen D.
Villa, Agnessa

Class 1953—Continued

Ward, Elizabeth (Mrs. Murray Plant)
Whitelaw, Mary E. (Mrs. W. G. Huxtable)
Williams, Susan F. (Mrs. D. M. Webster)
Wilson, Muriel (Mrs. Wilson Skaalen)
Younie, Jean L. (Mrs. Wm. R. S. Hardy)

Class 1954

Bacon, Joyce
Bishop, Janet
Berwanger, Ann (Mrs. Russell Mullan)
Brunlees, Donna M.
Burt, Elaine
Candlish, Marjorie G.
Cassidy, Audrey L. (Mrs. Herbert Renwick)
Clark, Norah E. (Mrs. Guy Beaudette)
Deacon, Jean M.
Dunk, Margaret B.
Dunsmore, Audrey A.
Edgecombe, E. Ann (Mrs. James B. King)
Fergus, Nora
Fraser, Lois A. (Mrs. James Parker)
Fuller, Hazel J. (Mrs. Charles E. Noel)
Gatehouse, Gloria
Gerrish, Harriet B. (Mrs. Eric B. Whynacht)
Gilbert, Ethel M. (Mrs. Carl Moore)
Goodfellow, Mary (Mrs. Gilbert Groome)
Greig, Helen (Mrs. R. E. Leigh)
Haliday, Alice (Mrs. John Walsh)
Harford, Sheila
Heslop, Ann M. E. (Mrs. Ann Findlay)
Harris, Lorna M. E. (Mrs. M. J. Brown)
Ingram, Ruth (Mrs. Ray McIntosh)
Irwin, Jane L. (Mrs. J. Einarson)
Loring, Anne E. (Mrs. A. Wadsworth)
Maguire, Rita (Mrs. Douglas Leach)
Marwick, E. Claire (Mrs. R. S. King)
Meredith, Marijean (Mrs. Ronald M. Major)
Mieszkowska, Krystyna O.
McDougall, Florence (Mrs. Kenneth Robinson)
McLean, A. Evelyn
MacMillan, Elizabeth L.
MacMillan, Sarah A. (Mrs. Murray MacDonald)
Nurse, Joan L. (Mrs. Ernest Tetreault)
Orr, T. Joan (Mrs. E. P. Smith)
Perkins, Myra J. (Mrs. R. D. Smith)
Perry, Phyllis
Preston, Jean (Mrs. McDaniel)
Renaud, A. Anne (Mrs. Allan McKay)
Robinson, Barbara
Rumsey, E. Irene
Ryan, Patricia
Saunderson, Eileen (Mrs. S. Vaudry)
Smith, Margaret K. (Mrs. A. C. S. Stead)
Stewart, Ardyth A.
Tanner, Patricia
Tyler, Marlene
Walker, Ann E.
Wilkinson, Joan D. (Mrs. D. M. Lewis)
Williams, Marjory M.
Wilson, Susan
Yates, M. Ruth

Class 1955

Allan, Barbara (Mrs. B. Mann)
Appleton, Louise (Mrs. John Zwirewich)
Armstrong, Isabel
Bulman, Sheila
Burton, Beverley (Mrs. C. H. Neale)
Bushell, M. Frances
Buzzell, Lorraine
Buzzell, Mary
Cameron, Joan (Mrs. James Wood)
Crawford, D. Ann (Mrs. Donald Lowering)
Cummings, Joan (Mrs. Donald B. McKnight)

Class 1955—Continued

Denovan, Audrey (Mrs. Donald Bellamy)
Dixon, Mary (Mrs. Arthur Williams)
Doherty, Elda (Mrs. A. S. Hackwell)
Dorken, Elaine
Duncan, Gladys (Mrs. Irvine Johnston)
Fitzpatrick, Janet (married)
Goodyear, Barbara (Mrs. Cecil Stein)
Hackwell, Joy
Hampson, M. Gay (Mrs. A. H. Speirs)
Hanson, Glenda (Mrs. A. Van Hoorn)
Harrison, Marion
Heron, Mary
Hewett, Joan
Hick, Carol (Mrs. C. A. Smith)
Hogg, Grace
Hohne, Gisela
Holmes, Barbara
Hooper, Mary Louise (Mrs. E. L. Buchanan)
Johnson, Phyllis (Mrs. Stuart B. Bruce)
Jordan, Margaret (Mrs. M. J. Nicoll-Griffith)
Lanctot, M. Beryll (Mrs. G. Laatunen)
Lay, Grace (Mrs. Howard Roach)
MacLeod, Dorothy (Mrs. Keith Drummond)
McMahon, Kathleen (Mrs. A. Meyer)
Mainwaring, Claire (Mrs. Howard O'Quinn)
Mitchell, Mary (Mrs. William Woodward)
Mornan, Margaret
Morris, Mavis (Mrs. Lindsay Smith)
Robb, Joan (Mrs. Alex. K. Paterson)
Ross, Sally (Mrs. Ingmar E. Larsson)
Sawyer, Doreen (Mrs. L. Acres)
Scott, Heather (Mrs. Peter Hall)
Shaw, Patricia (Mrs. K. G. Menear)
Sheltus, Kathryn
Sohn, Ana Luisa (Mrs. P. E. Maigler)
Trebilcock, Ruth (Mrs. Ian Gilbert)
Turnbull, Freda
Valdstyn, Alena
Walkington, B. Jane (Mrs. Richard C. Rokeby)
Wellein, Mary (Mrs. Robert H. Thicke)
Winser, Shirley (Mrs. E. C. Durocher)

Class 1956

Allison, Jane (Mrs. Robert Hayward)
Auger, Jacquelyn (Mrs. Ian Gray)
Beattie, Janice
Bergeron, Lise (Mrs. D. Stewart)
Bown, Patricia (Mrs. J. D. Giegerich)
Bryant, Constance (Mrs. R. C. Allen)
Brostyan, Esther (Mrs. Philip Hamelin)
Brown, Barbara
Burnett, Ishbel (Mrs. H. Grauer)
Charles, Audrey (Mrs. M. Bolton)
Coulthard, Anne (Mrs. R. B. Hokea)
Currier, Catherine (Mrs. G. R. Francis)
Elger, Lorna (Mrs. P. C. MacIntosh)
Estey, Margaret (Mrs. R. Whalen)
Forneret, Elizabeth
Gauthier, Madeleine
Gilmour, Mary
Gold, Nancy
Grant, Joan (Mrs. Desmond McCauley)
Henderson, Viola (Mrs. Carl M. Glos)
Hewetson, Patricia E. (Mrs. J. C. Meyer)
Hunter, Freda
Kuehn, Patricia
Larnder, Eve
Lochead, Elizabeth
Malone, Maureen
Marler, Susan
McColm, Katherine (Mrs. Ian Wilson)
Newberg, Joanne Louise (Mrs. D. W. Argall)
Noel, Winnifred (Mrs. J. Butterfield)
Page, Joyce (Mrs. Basile Sevriuk)
Pattison, Moira (Mrs. Emile Kanim)

Class 1956—Continued

Pennell, Joan
Persurich, Anna
Pick, Vera
Plomer, Marley
Rowley, Helen Anne
Saunders, Joyce (Mrs. Richard Schulz)
Seeley, Evelyn (Mrs. R. F. Irvine)
Smith, Audrey (Mrs. F. Shackell)
Stearns, Evelyne (Mrs. Paul Murphy)
Stewart, Grace (Mrs. D. S. Crowell)
Strike, Eileen
Sumner, Joan (Mrs. Berand deKat)
Turner, Ann
Underhill, Olive (Mrs. O. Andrasi)
Walker, Susanne (Mrs. John Green)
Webster, Patricia
Zajac, Nadia (Mrs. J. A. D'Urso)

Class 1957

Aboud, Viola
Anderson, Heather J. (Mrs. A. Thuswaldner)
Bailey, Ruth E. (Mrs. Eric Stackhouse)
Bain, Beverley A.
Bangs, Mary (Mrs. M. Watson)
Beattie, Nancy L. (Mrs. John Price)
Benaim, Fay
Best, Marie Louise (Mrs. R. D. Westervelt)
Binns, Patricia
Bishop, Mary Ann
Boelen, Elizabeth V. (Mrs. L. J. Emond)
Bond, Mary I. (Mrs. R. Matte)
Brewer, Helen J. (Mrs. John E. McCombe)
Butters, Jean M. (Mrs. K. G. O'Brien)
Cummings, Elizabeth (Mrs. F. W. Irwin)
Davis, Patricia (Mrs. J. E. Miller)
Drennan, Marilyn (Mrs. Ronald S. Snow)
Fawthrop, June S.
Freeman, Shirley (Mrs. P. J. Vanier)
Gerrie, Susan D. (Mrs. N. J. Buka)
Gilder, Josephine
Hannen, Helen F. (Mrs. Gabriel White)
Haughn, Janice B. (Mrs. Albert Morgan)
Horner, Grace S. (Mrs. R. W. Wilson)
Hunter, Nancy L. (Mrs. J. A. Sosa)
Hume, Sara
Jackson, Elizabeth A.
Jefferys, Louise
Jervis, Margaret A. (Mrs. John L. Carson)
Johnson, Helen C.
Lawson, Margaret E. (Mrs. Kaye Huet)
LePot, Doreen
McCormick, Nancy
McDonald, Marion
MacDonald, Kathleen L. (Mrs. F. H. Rasmussen)
McKean, Carol (Mrs. J. W. Isaac)
MacLean, Shirley I. (Mrs. David W. Bailey)
MacLeod, Barbara J. (Mrs. Michael D. Arthur)
McCabe, Carol J. (Mrs. D. Hogg)
McCutcheon, Roberta M.
McLaughlin, M. M. A. Louise (Mrs. Wm. J. Kalaher)
McQuarrie, Margaret (Mrs. E. L. McCallum)
McVety, Ann E.
Mitchell, Jane Ellen
Mountain, Mary V. (Mrs. Harry Parker)
Neil, Marion (Mrs. M. Barnard)
Page, Mary Denise
Pepler, Carolyn J.
Philips, Dorothy A. M.
Pond, Joan H.
Price, Willa
Quinlan, Janet E.
Rasmussen, Inge M.
Reaper, Carol (Mrs. F. Morrison)
Reed, Sarah (Mrs. M. R. Hodgson)

Class 1957—Continued

Ritchie, Sylvia O.
Roach, Barbara (Mrs. Vollen Hastings)
Rutherford, Andrea (Mrs. J. H. Burgess)
Sargent, Priscilla
Saunders, Doris
Saunders, Joan N. (Mrs. Charles Freedman)
Scott, Carolyn M. (Mrs. Lorne Ingham)
Searle, Mary
Shirley, Maudrene S. (Mrs. Gordon Butters)
Simpson, Carol A. (Mrs. Daniel Pitt)
Smallwood, Maryjean (Mrs. M. McCory)
Stephenson, Margaret G.
Stowe, Constance M.
Sullivan, Catherine E.
Takacs, Pearl
Talbot, Mary (Mrs. Ian Lundie)
Thompson, Mary E. (Mrs. M. R. Scriven)
Thompson, Virginia I.
Tyler, Ainslie (Mrs. T. P. Webster)
Wathen, Mary (Mrs. Wm. P. Keating)
White, Shirley W.
Woodcock, Ann Elizabeth (Mrs. J. A. Gray)

Class 1958

Aird, Judith A.
Barnes, Barbara E.
Bennett, Joan Lillian
Black, L. Joyce (Mrs. R. Hicklin)
Boland, Veronica L. (Mrs. N. Valentine)
Bradbury, Ruth E. (Mrs. Kenneth Henderson)
Bragger, Elizabeth Carole (Mrs. R. L. Purdy)
Burkhardt, Mildred J.
Cerry, Ann L. (Mrs. Paul A. Davis)
Chagnon, Jeannine R.
Clements, Jane Elizabeth (Mrs. J. Donaldson)
Colquhoun, Anne I. (Mrs. A. Mines)
Cooke, Helen E.
Cousens, Margaret R.
Cowie, Margaret E.
Crook, Marilyn A.
Diplock, M. Linda (Mrs. Ross J. Collie)
Doupe, Carolyn M.
Drew, Sara Louise (Mrs. R. B. Cope)
Edwards, Terrill Joan (Mrs. W. T. Pittman)
Fisk, Dorothy A. (Mrs. Gerald Durant)
French, Terrill Joan (Mrs. W. T. Pittman)
George, Patricia A.
Gould, H. E. Aileen (Mrs P. E. Carlson)
Gray, Catherine A.
Griffith, Eunice Irene
Guest, Norah A.
Haldimand, Carol Ann (Mrs. F. Steele)
Hall, Margaret Monica
Hanna, Barbara A. (Mrs. David H. Bush)
Hastings, Beverley J. (Mrs. James McBride)
Hawkins, Mary Joan Roberts (Mrs. J. Fagan)
Hendry, Joan P. (Mrs. G. E. Norman)
Hill, Dorothy J.
Hooper, Frances Elizabeth
Horning, Sharon I.
Hulbert, P. Ann (Mrs. P. Morrison)
Hutchison, Sandra Mary (Mrs. W. E. Arute)
Jeffrey, Carole J. G. (Mrs. J. Maynard)
Johnson, Diana G. (Mrs. David M. Hunter)
King, Lorna Aileen (Mrs. Gordon E. Purdy)
Laing, Alexandra J. (Mrs. David G. Hogg)
Le Heron, Evelyn Sylvania
Lemon, Louise (Mrs. H. Curtis)
Little, Sandra (Mrs. John F. Cameron)
Logan, Sandra Mikell (Mrs. Kenneth Scott)
Lyn, Yvonne Eloise
McCallum, Mary E.
Mackenzie, Heather M.
MacLean, Sheila Anne (Mrs. R. K. Seaman)
MacMillan, Marion Jessie

APPENDIX C

Class 1958—Continued

Martin, Pauline I.
Moersfelder, Margaret Elenora (Mrs. John Waldhouser)
Moll, Barbara R.
Mornan, Elizabeth Ann (Mrs. E. A. Noble)
Murphy, S. A. Eileen
Nielsen, Edna (Mrs. J. P. Schell)
Norton, Margaret M. (Mrs. M. Malboeuf)
O'Brien, Lois Ann (Mrs. C. Ashton)
Oram, Diane Edith (Mrs. Bruce N. Harper)
Pearce, Elizabeth M.
Peters, Margaret Jean
Ponthieu, D. Phyllis (Mrs. Peter Anastasides)
Prentice, Marilyn E.
Pye, Nancy-Lee
Reynolds, Sybil Ann (Mrs. Ross M. Southwood)
Richards, Elizabeth A. (Mrs. John Edge)
Ritchie, Janice A. (Mrs. Gerald Cousens)
Rossiter, Marilyn (Mrs. Peter Clark)
Schippel, Sandra C. (Mrs. Ross T. Sykes)
Scott, Dorothy Eleanor
Shoofey, Patricia Mary B.
Shurly, Virginia J.
Snidal, Ellen S. (Mrs. Garth E. Mosher)
Soper, Marie-Helene-Ethel (Mrs. R. Freeman)
Stewart, Barbara
Stewart, Catherine A.
Strange, M. Jane (Mrs. John L. Fisher)
Theriault, Lorraine Jocelyn
Thompson, Linda L. (Mrs. R. A. MacLeod)
Thurber, Mary Josephine F.
Tippett, Jo-Ann Elizabeth (Mrs. J. Fox)
Tomaschuk, Elaine H. (Mrs. Kenneth Steels)
Tweedy, Katherine Jean (Mrs. Rodger Perry)
Tyszkiewicz, Ronia M. T.
Velisek, A. Hemma (Mrs. Douglas C. Fraser)
Walsh, Patricia (Mrs. P. Bowering)
Welsh, Carol Ann
Whittaker, Patricia A. (Mrs. I. Nielsen)
Wilson, Shirley Joan (Mrs. Terrence Gregory)
Wood, Nancy Eleanor (Mrs. R. Roy)
Woods, Ann Elizabeth (Mrs. R. F. Bertrand)

Class 1959

Anderson, Mary Marjorie
Arnold, Dorothy Marguerite Kay
Beeman, Kathleen Russell
Berger, Maria
Biggs, Lois Ann (Mrs. Richard Ogilvy)
Briard, Heather Ann
Bray, Dale (Mrs. A. J. Hall)
Burke, Barbara Eve
Campbell, Florence Jeffers (Mrs. J. S. Redpath)
Chamberlain, Kathryn Gayle (Mrs. G. A. Boire)
Clark, Joan Margaret Mabel
Clark, Beverley Anne Marie (Mrs. Wm. N. Caldwell)
Connor, Carole D.
Cornfield, Margaret (Mrs. R. Quesnelles)
Creighton, E. Ann (Mrs. W. A. Buik)
Cummer, Beverley Gail (Mrs. J. E. Gelety)
Currie, Marion Joan
Cuthbertson, Maude Suzanne
Davies, Noreen Beverley
Dazé, Laura Ann
Dewar, Barbara Eileen
Dey, Shirley Elizabeth (Mrs. S. Captain)
Dentremont, Judith (Mrs. D. Taylor)
Dorion, Doreen (Mrs. J. O'Brien)
Dwyer, Joan (Mrs. James H. McNeil)
Ellicott, Ann
Ferris, Evelyn Marie
Forth, Mary Elizabeth
Gagnon, Carol Anne Mabe
Gagnon, Rose Mary
Gillingham, Grace Beverley (Mrs. D. Currie)

Class 1959—Continued

Glasheen, Joan
Gourlay, Glenda Ellen
Hague, Florence Elizabeth
Hall, Agnes Beverley
Hambly, Barbara Louise
Hartley, Margaret Ellen (Mrs. R. A. Hango)
Haslam, Margaret Marilyn
Hickey, Beverley (Mrs. John Lough)
Hill, Diana
Hodges, Barbara Seaton (Mrs. J. R. Parker)
Holton, Heather Symington
Hornibrook, Mary Elaine (Mrs. Wm. McRae)
Jeffrey, Dawn Heather (married)
Jeffrey, Lois Margo
Johnston, Robin Alexandra
Kennedy, Margaret (Mrs. M. Bragger)
Kerr, Elizabeth Mary (Mrs. Bruce Watt)
Krumm, Nina Frances (Mrs. Lewis Winter)
Lahue, Janice Kathleen
Lang, Sally Jane (Mrs. John Kaye)
Lunam, Rosemary (Mrs. Keith F. McLeary)
Lussier, Irene
Magnan, Rose Marie (Mrs. R. A. Marentette)
Major, Elizabeth Winnifred (Mrs. C. C. B. Wilson)
Mark, Barbara Ann
Martin, Carole (Mrs. Derek Dempster)
Matschen, Ursula
Mattern, Shirley Joan (Mrs. W. A. Kilpatrick)
Moore, Angela Claire
Mowry, Lynne (Mrs. M. A. Ashworth)
MacBeth, Margaret Elizabeth
MacCallum, Heather (Mrs. K. C. Ashline)
MacKay, Laura Wells
MacLeod, Shirley
MacLeod, Velma
MacMillan, Sheila Mary (Mrs. Edgar L. Darling)
McEvoy, Barbara Ann
McGee, Anna Mary Kathleen
McKinnon, Anita Claire
McKinnon, Janice Eleanor
Naylor, Rachel Clare (Mrs. Ronald Fletcher)
Nelson, Elizabeth
Newington, Isabel
Newell, Barbara Jane (Mrs. John S. Auston)
Nicholson, Betsy
Nisbet, Doreen Olive
Owens, Margaret
Pratt, Isabelle Marcia (Mrs. Wm. G. MacDonald)
Preston, Patricia Renfrew
Randall, Katherine Margaret
Redfern, Maureen Worsley (Mrs. Julian H. Huxham)
Reynolds, Margaret Stroud (Mrs. Hugo Grout)
Roberts, Carol Margaret
Roberts, Judith Scott Ferguson
Ross, Margaret May (Mrs. R. Le Maitre)
Rudinsky, Ann (Mrs. John Smarzik)
Rzemien, Stephanie Rosali
Sadler, Margaret Elizabeth
Salmon, Nedra
Sault, Kathryn Anne
Schneider, Hana Viviane (Mrs. James C. Ashfield)
Sewell, Janet Emily
Sheppard, Helen (Mrs. C. W. Walker)
Simpson, Heather May
Sinclair, Jean (Mrs. James M. Donnell)
Skroder, Gail Marena (Mrs. Brian Mosgrave)
Smith, Mary Julia
Smith, Mary Jane Margaret
Smith, Helen Beverley (Mrs. Hector McInnes)
Smith, Nancy Jane
Stenson, Gail Margaret
Stephenson, Claire Gilmour
Stevens, Judith Louise
Strang, Barbara Ann

Class 1959—Continued

Strang, Marilyn Jean (Mrs. R. P. Bates)
Strom, Margery Victoria
Thurston, Ann (Mrs. Alister M. Ingram)
Vance, Clara Letitia
Waller, Iris (Mrs. Robert B. Bisson)
Werrett, Marilyn Rose
Wilkinson, Doris Elizabeth
Wilson, Dorothy Mary (Mrs. Claude Papineau)
Wilson, Kathleen Margaret
Wittenborn, Gillian Joyce
Zmroczek, Agnes

Class 1960

Bentley, Carol Ann
Bethune, Joyce Eillen
Bieber, Barbara Ann (Mrs. P. Kessler)
Borkovich, Miriam Annie (Mrs. F. McManus)
Bowle-Evans, Wendy
Boyle, Barbara Joan
Buchanan, Carol Edwina
Butler, Patricia Ann (Mrs. J. K. Riches)
Castle, Kathleen Winona (Mrs. W. Richardson)
Connor, Audrey E. Anne
Currie, Davena Helen (Mrs. H. R. Bailey)
Dallas, Sandra Mary
Dallison, Jean Olga
Davis, Marjorie J. (Mrs. R. Dendy)
Dore, Jessie Barbara
Droeske, Patricia Ruth
Dunlop, Cynthia deBlois (Mrs. D. G. Hicks)
Eldridge, Margaret Susan
Elliot, Joan Stewart (Mrs. T. Miller)
Estey, Catherine G.
Evans, Patricia E.
Flemming, Jane Irene
Fraser, Catherine Elizabeth
Gartshore, Annis May
Gelinas, Marilyn Edna (Mrs. R. E. Page)
Gillespie, Barbara Ellenor
Goddard, Lynn Doris
Gow, Christina McPhail
Hamlin, Sigrid Joan (Mrs. John D. Tolmie)
Harrison, Lynne Adair
Helm, Dorothy Evelyn
Juno, Carol Barbara
Kee, Sandra Brittain
Kerr, Phyllis Margaret
Labey, Ann Wynifred A. (Mrs. K. Clements)
Leinonen, Norma Lois
Leutbecher, Hannah Elise
Lewis, Geraldine Elizabeth
Lyman, Deirdre Suzanne
MacLean, Barbara Constance
MacTier, Margaret Joan (Mrs. K. Tricky)
Marchuk, Carol Marlene (married)
McCraw, Margaret M. M. (Mrs. T. Riley)
McDonald, Margaret P. Anne
Martin, Joan Evelyn D.
Miles, Donna Kathleen (Mrs. S. Vaughan)
Montgomery, Nancy Elizabeth
Nettleship, June Gertrude (Mrs. J. Carson)
Nicholas, Penelope Dawn
Nourse, Nancy Grace
Nunan, Gail Maureen K.
Paget, Anne Dorothy
Piercey, Celia Joan (Mrs. L. Fisher)
Rerrie, Annabel Louise
Robertson, Jane Taylor
Shaw, Diane (Mrs. H. G. Scott)
Singlehurst, Jane Arden
Smith, Angela Mary
Smith, Rosemary Doris W. (Mrs. R. Campbell)
Stevens, Myrna Dale
Sumner, Mary Frances
Thomson, Corinne Patricia (Mrs. D. Carnegie)
Thornton, Lynda Bronwyn

Class 1960—Continued

Turnbull, Dorothy Jane
Turner, Sadie Payne
Walcot, Marguerite Alice
Wright, Eileen Patricia
Yates, Berta Essie Jane
Young, Patricia Ann
Zawadski, Anna (Mrs. W. Stachmyk)

Class 1961

Anderson, Betty Lou
Ardagh, Diana Marie (Mrs. George Elias)
Ashworth, Judith Mary
Ball, Ruth Charlotte
Barlow, Andrea
Barnhart, Leslie Ann
Beal, Georgiana Kathleen
Berladyn, Barbara Olga
Bowering, Jacqueline
Burke, Barbara Marie
Burwash, Nancy
Calder, Roberta Jean
Charles, Mary Vernon Hughes
Church, Diana Mary
Clark, Margaret Rose
Clark, Suzanne
Cloghesy, Helen Theresa
Colgan, Mary Elizabeth
Croft, Jean Alice
Crutchfield, Constance Mae (Mrs. G. S. Scott)
Deeley, Margaret Anne
Dobson, Barbara Lee
Donnan, Sheila Jean
Downey, Sandra Audrey
Du Vernet, Wendy Mary
Eggertson, Jona Laurelle
Farnsworth, Gwenyth Ann
Farquharson, Penelope Courtenay
Feeney, Joanne
Fitz Gerald, Noreen Elsa
Fitzpatrick, Audrey Lois
Francis, Margaret Lynne
Fraser, Andrea Jean
Gascoigne, Dawn Eleanor
Gillies, Nancy Ann
Girvan, Mary Douglas
Goodeve, Jill Elizabeth
Greene, Arlene Carole
Grosvalet, Helen Marion
Hair, Helen Lynne
Hall, Ann Jean Elizabeth
Hanna, Noel Jane
Harnum, Elizabeth Jacqueline
Harper, Jane Isabel
Hassinger, Janet Ann Veronica
Heward, Beverley Frances
Jackson, Susan Erica
Jenkins, Jill Caroline F.
Johnstone, Margaret Anne
Jones, Sheila Gwendolyn
Joyce, Carolyn Anne
Keith, Mary Helen
Kent, Margaret Rosalie (Mrs. B. T. Smith)
Kerr, Donna
Kerr, Judith Doreen
Lake, Jane Anne
Lamb, Barbara Joan
Lennon, Margaret Jane
Lockwood, Patricia
MacGregor, Jean Anne (Mrs. R. P. Elliott)
Malcolmson, Ann Elizabeth
Mansfield, Barbara Elizabeth
Mason, Mary Linda
McKenzie, Carroll Diane
McKinnon, Katherine Lyle
McLaughlin, Kathleen

Class 1961—Continued

McNeill, Sheila Elizabeth
Mellor, Margaret Ruth
Memory, Marilyn Ann
Meredith, Dorothy Diane P.
Millican, Brenda J. (Jan)
Molyneux, Joan
Murray, Anne Ruth
Neil, Myrna Elizabeth
Norton, Eileen Dorothy
O'Boyle, Marsha Johanne
Ohman, Audrey Jean Murray
Palmer, Dorothy Claudette
Pollock, Shirley A. M.
Quigg, Maureen Gwendolyn
Robison, Andrea Claire
Rollock, Maureen Angelia
Ross, Kathleen Mary
Ross, Nancy Elizabeth
Salat, Eleanor Florence
Schindler, Carol Gail
Silver, Corinne Allyn

Class 1961—Continued

Smith, Helen Maud
Snyder, Helen Stewart
Stansfield, Patricia Anne
Stanton, Shirley Eleanor
Stewart, Barbara Lois
Tannahill, Faith
Taylor, Beverley Mackin
Taylor, Daphne Gwendolyn
Trebichavsky, Nadezda Eva (Nadia)
Vaughan, Barbara Ann
Waldock, Hilary Wenden
Walker, Helen Isabel
Webster, Nena Rosalind
Weeks, Linda Susan
West, Jo-Anne Merle (Mrs. Daniel Scholz)
Whalen, Gloria Mona
White, Helen Catherine
Wilson, Evelyn Gay
Winter, Marion L. (Marlo)
Woodman, Gail Stevens
Wyman, Margaret Elizabeth

GRADUATES OF THE WESTERN HOSPITAL

Class 1889
Beauchamp, Minnie (deceased)
Greece, K. (married) (deceased)
Moody, Irene (married) (deceased)
Nelson, J.

Class 1890
Bradley, M. (deceased)
Deacon, Ethel (deceased)
McGregor, C. A. (deceased)

Class 1891
Thompson, Bella (deceased)

Class 1892
Beauchamp, Emily (deceased)

Class 1893
Harriet-Bissett, J. B. (deceased)
Sixby, L. M. (deceased)
Wright, Mrs. Wm.

Class 1894
Hooper, M. (deceased)
Lewis, A. T. (deceased)
McBeath, Fanny (deceased)
Parker, H. F. (Mrs. H. Langley)
Pemberton, E.

Class 1895
Gilman, Elsie
Hill, Dora
Picken, A. (Mrs. J. Kerr)
Talmage, E.
Taylor, J. (deceased)

Class 1896
Bates, M.D. (Mrs. Davidson)
Fiske, H. (deceased)
Lawrence, S. W. (Mrs. S. Kerr) (deceased)
McLean, Sara (Mrs. K. McLean)

Class 1897
Potter-Smith, Mrs.

Class 1898
Harvey, E.
England, E. (married) (deceased)

Class 1899
Kent, (Mrs. Stobie)
Miller, R. J.
Reinhardt, M. (deceased)
Stuart, B.A. (Mrs. A. Taylor)

Class 1900
Clauston, E. M.
Johnson, A.

Class 1901
Davies, C. J. (deceased)

Class 1902
Byers, E. H.
Hodgson, E. (married)
Keddie, J. V.
McKeand, H. H.
Murphy, A. (married)

Class 1903
Bates, E.
Bostwick, B.
Byers, J. T.
Canovan, O. (deceased)
Devine, L.
Diplock, E. (married)
Hughes, A. (Mrs. R.Cleary) (deceased)
Lewis, E.
Sullivan, E.
Vance, A. (deceased)
Whitney, H. (Mrs. R. Wilson)

Class 1904
Griffiths, Mrs. E.
Gryce, L. (Mrs. Wright)
Hull, H. (deceased)
McKinnon, J. O. (Mrs. Baker)
Mathews, O. (Mrs. Geo. Briggs)

Class 1905

Anderson, J.
Campbell, E. M.
Cleland, A. (deceased)
Geddes, I. F. (married)
Hector, J. (Mrs. E. Donnelly)
Hunter, M.
Lecouter, G. (Mrs. G. B. Wenzel)
Leslie, M.
Loggie, E. B. (married)
MacDonald F. (deceased)
Munro, M.

Class 1906

Aitken, A. A.
Gretchell, A. E. (Mrs. Brush)
Munn, Rosa (married)
Wright, E. A. (deceased)

Class 1907

Bennett, Leeta (Mrs. E. Butson)
Cameron, Margaret J. (Mrs. Watson Austen Constable)
Hall, Lena V. (Mrs. MacMillan)
Hippen, Katherine (Mrs. Campbell)
McArthur, Jean (deceased)
Morrison, Marion F.
Noseworthy, H. A. (deceased)
Turner, E. Maud (Mrs. J. Rose)
Wilson, Dorothy M. (Mrs. C. H. Hamilton)
(deceased)

Class 1908

Bucken, B. (Mrs. J. Smeaton)
Flynn, Anita T.
MacDonell, Anna (Mrs. Bond) (deceased)
MacLean, Ethel (Mrs. G. H. Stewart)

Class 1909

Eaman, Ethel
Wilkinson, Ada

Class 1910

Alexander, Bessie A. (Mrs. I. Jones)
Bates, Edna M. (Mrs. Jas. Franckum)
Burns, Edith
Dougherty, Beatrice (Mrs. A. P. Bond)
Douglas, Grace (Mrs. J. Russell)
Drake, Mabel R.
Jennings, Isobel (deceased)
Keech, Elizabeth (deceased)
Kennedy, Gwendolyn (Mrs. A. Raymond)
Maw, S. Gertrude (Mrs. C. E. Horsman)
Nash, Marion
Pickel, Muriel E. (Mrs. J. V. Owens)
Scriver, Mary August (Mrs. J. R. Tait)
Wiggett, Clara G.

Class 1911

Coyle, M. Eileen (Mrs. A. J. Hebert)
Finigan, M. Matilda
Gerard, Grace
Grimson, Ellen C. (deceased)
Gunn, Elva
Hinde, Elizabeth (Mrs. J. B. Carswell)
MacGregor, Lillian C. (Mrs. Lloyd Scott)
Moore, M. Lena
Perreault, Emily M.
Snow, Alice M. (Mrs. F. R. Phenix)
Telling, Maude (deceased)

Class 1912

Birch, Bertha
Donnelly, Evelyn (Mrs. G. Couglan)
Dyer, Beatrice A.
McCall, Mary
McCleverty, Lydia (Mrs. C. T. Bradshaw)
Nicol, Ethel (deceased)
Salmon, Florence (deceased)
Ward, Daisy (Mrs. A. H. C. Carson)
Wilson, Jessie

Class 1913

Cooper, Eleanor (Mrs. Harry Wallace)
Crossley, Emile H. (deceased)
Corby, Ethel S. (deceased)
Ellis, Eleanor
McAllister, Carolyn
Rankin, Helen (married) (deceased)
Reveler, Mabel (Mrs. McKeracher)
Shepherd, Ada
Stratton, Jean H.
Wiggett, Kathleen W. (Mrs. H. Shepherd)

Class 1914

Argue, Ella A. (Mrs. Takaberry)
Armstrong, Muriel (Mrs. B. L. Wickware)
Benton, Emmeline (Mrs. A. Penny)
Bradley, Ethel F.
DeLacy, Marie (Mrs. E. D. Brown)
Doherty, Mary Helen (Mrs. G. E. Dingle)
Etherington, Edythe
Gallagher, Edith A. (Mrs. Kerr)
Graham, Mary
Leavitt, Margaret (Mrs. S. Morrison)
Logan, Rhoda (Mrs. Finley Monro)
McRae, Margaret B. (Mrs. Howard Clouston)
(deceased)
McRae, Pearl
McWhirter, Evelyn
Nixon, Charlotte
Reynar, Mabel, A.R.R.C.

Class 1915

Cuthbertson, Hilda (deceased)
Dean, Phyllis (Mrs. M. C. Small)
Lotto, Mary Louise
McCombe, Mildred A. (Mrs. N. G. B. Allan)
McLeod, Bessie (deceased)
Morrison, Mary Ethel
Stark, Deborah B. (Mrs. C. B. Gamsby)
Stevens, Doris M.
Yeats, Annie G.

Class 1916

Charlton, E. M. (Mrs. Allan Gammell)
Chisnolm, Ada (Mrs. Harold Pope)
Hume, Margaret
McDonald, Alexandra
Robertson, Ruth M.
Robertson, Irene F. (Mrs. H. McLean)
Raymond, Ella (Mrs. Gordon McNaughton)
Sutton, Lucy E.
Tessier, Ruby A. (Mrs. Lewis Smith)
Williams, Harriet
Whitehead, Mary (Mrs. H. McDougall)

Class 1917

Brand, Lillian
Clough, Lena (Mrs. DeSantos)
Collins, M. Maud (Mrs. A. D. Buchanan)

Class 1917—Continued

Cunningham, Isabel G. (Mrs. John Anderson)
    (deceased)
Fowles, Mabel C. (Mrs. Wm. Daw)
Green, Mabel V. (Mrs. Colin C. Barclay)
Halford, J. Margaret (Mrs. Miller)
Hartley, Eleanor F. (Mrs. G. S. Lemasnie)
    (deceased)
McKee, Edith M. (Mrs. R. Cariss)
Moore, Julia B. (Mrs. Argue)
Morency, Beatrice B. (Mrs. W. H. Hill)
Rowley, Christina H. (Mrs. P. Robertson)

Class 1918

Cunningham, Eileen (Mrs. C. C. Rathe)
Davison, Evelyn (Mrs. J. J. Pollock)
Hill, Bessie G.
Leavitt, Ruth M. (deceased)
Mount, Ethel E. (Mrs. J. B. Chalk)
Payne, Edna I.
Platt, Mabel (Mrs. Thos. Littlejohns)
Ross, Edythe S. M. (married)
Stephens, Avelina M. (Mrs. Gordon Anderson)
Telfer, Jessie J. (Mrs. Albert Wasson)
Watson, Marjorie (Mrs. Jas. Craig) (deceased)
Whimby, Elizabeth M.

Class 1919

Barr, Estelle (deceased)
Cameron, Sarah (Mrs. A. Kennedy)
Charlton, Winnifred M. (Mrs. Roy)
Fawcett, Mattie (Mrs. E. C. Copping)
Hooper, Daisy (Mrs. Wm. Hunter)
McNie, Florence (Mrs. R. Pennoyer) (deceased)
Reyner, Marjorie B.
Taylor, Doris (Mrs. R. J. Inglis)
Wright, Pansy B.

Class 1920

Brain, Dorothy (Mrs. H. S. Windeler)
Chisholm, Hanna
Cornell, Gladys I (Mrs. Leslie Roberts)
Damon, Fanny E.
Hamilton, E. Grace
Kelly, Katherine
Muir, Edna
Robertson, Vivienne M. (Mrs. N. E. Fletcher)
MacWhinnie, Myrtle
Wheeler, Dorothy G. (married)

Class 1921

Armitage, Frances (Mrs. R. Rowley)
Barrett, Mary E.
Beckstead, Marion (Mrs. M. Gillespie)
Fowles, Eleanor G. (Mrs. J. B. Caldwell)
Gagnon, Louise
Kerr, Hazel
LeHuray, Olive H. (Mrs. R. Bray)
Phelan, Una M. (Mrs. W. V. Bartlett)
Winton, Margaret H.

Class 1922

Brain, Elsie
Gillespie, Marion A.
Jackson, Ada G. (Mrs. Strickland) (deceased)
Johnston, Marguerite
Johnson, Lillian

Class 1922—Continued

Lilly, Olga (Mrs. A. O. Barwick)
Lucas, Viola May
Martin, Florence S.
McLaughlin, Laura M.
Murray, Margaret
Savage, B.
Scullin, Anne (Mrs. F. Murphy)
Winnall, Stella H. (Mrs. Angus Barwick)

Class 1923

Barnes, Kathleen (Mrs. C. Boyce)
Crawford, Phoebe
Farrar, Phyllis B. (Mrs. Norman Rothwell)
Gear, Beatrice M.
Jacques, Beatrice M.
Martin, M. Grace (deceased)
Sharp, Mary Ella (Mrs. H. A. Palmer)
Taylor, Christina S.
Tyrrell, Margaret L.

Class 1924

Bates, Edna A.
Bouresk, Alexandra (Mrs. R. Stewart)
Butlan, Ellen R. (Mrs. Geo. Hume) (deceased)
Costigan, Agnes
Hooper, Eleanor M.
James, Freda M.
MacDonald, Flora (Mrs. MacDonald)
McCallum, Margaret E.
McClements, Mary M. (Mrs. Farrington)
Payne, Madeleine B. (Mrs. F. Beal)
Robinson, Mabel K. (married)
Smith, Hilda M.
Taggart, Mrs. Grace A. M.
Wintle, Cora H. (Mrs. Carl Brock)

Class 1925

Bates, E. Stella (Mrs. Heasham)
Black, Edith Harriet (Mrs. F. Hambly)
Corbett, Edna A.
Cunningham, Kathleen W.
Hanlon, Elizabeth
Hooper, Edith G. (Mrs. R. D. Thompson)
Kennedy, Mary F. (Mrs. R. Binks)
Kett, Ruby E. (Mrs. Rogers)
Munro, Margaret G.
Reynolds, Alexandra M.
Spier, Margaret M.
Whimbey, Florence C. (Mrs. R. K. Anderson)
Whimbey, Hazel Jean
White, Elizabeth R. (Mrs. Matheson)

Class 1926

Bryne, Maude E. (Mrs. R. D. King)
Carpenter, Rotha M. (deceased)
Clark, Cora M.
Cross, Violet A.
Harding, Aimee D. (Mrs. G. E. Riley)
Kerr, Vernie L.
MacFarlane, Margaret L. (Mrs. F. W. Bradshaw)
McCormick, Charlotte J. (Mrs. D. Sutherland)
McCrudden, Olga M.
McElroy, Margaret A. (Mrs. R. H. Morewood)
McOuat, Amy M. (Mrs. G. F. Calder) (deceased)
McPhee, Pernella (Mrs. Wm. Baldwin)
O'Reilly, Hilda H. (Mrs. G. W. Kelly)
Payn, Lillian E.

APPENDIX D

GRADUATE NURSES WHO SERVED OVERSEAS

WORLD WAR I – 1914-1918

Edith S. Anderson
Christine Arnoldi, A.R.R.C.
Helen Arnoldi
Beatrice Armitage
Pearl Babbit
Esthaol Bagshaw
F. Winnifred Brown
Harriet E. Carman
Lillian Carter
Edith Casswell
Margaret Christie
M. Birkett Clark
Evadne K. Cotter, A.R.R.C.
Alice Cooper
Marion Cole
Jennie L. Colburn
Isabel Davies, A.R.R.C.
Millicent Alice Day
Flora Dalgleish
E. Jane Dewar
Gertrude Decou
Lillian Dickie
Dorothy Downes
Jennette F. Duncan
Minnie E. Engelke, A.R.R.C.
Mildred H. Forbes, R.R.C.
Margaret Fortescue
Cicely Galt, A.R.R.C.
Clare Gass
Margaret A. Gillespie
Edna Giffen
Louella Gillis
Roberta Gourlay
Lilly Gray, A.R.R.C.
Janie B. Graham
E. Hestor Hardinge, A.R.R.C.
Frances A. Harnum
Eleanor Handcock
Sophie Hoerner, R.R.C.
Laura Holland, A.R.R.C.
Isabel Hobkirk
Harriet Hutchins
Idella A. Ingraham
Dora Jones
Elizabeth Kennedy
Kathleen M. Knight
Louisa Lanktree
Violet Larter
Lily Larter
Ruth Loggie
Mary V. Lovering
Georgina Massy

Jane E. Mann
Minnie Mitchell
Beatrice A. Moores
Anne Morewood
Dorothy B. Moss
Marie Muir
Mary L. MacDermot
Stella MacDougall
Olive A. Mackay, A.R.R.C.
Charlotte S. MacNaughton
Rachel McConnell, A.R.R.C.
Louise McGreer, A.R.R.C.
Louise F. McLeod
Katherine McLeod, A.R.R.C.
Mary W. McLeod
Helen M. McMurrich, Croix de Guerre
Helen Nelson, A.R.R.C.
Elizabeth Odell, R.R.C.
Bernice Outterson
Mary Orr
Gertrude M. Paget
Juliette Pelletier
Florence Perry
Jean T. Ramsay
Dorothy Rhodes
Winnie C. Riddle
Charlotte I. Robinson
Harriet M. Ross
Elizabeth B. Ross, R.R.C.
Marjorie Ross
Violet Sampson
Gladys Sare
Agnes Sargeant
Nina F. Sharp
Bertha A. Smith
Myrtle Stevens
Annie Jane Stevens
Constance Stuart
Isabella Strathy, A.R.R.C.
Annette Tate, A.R.R.C.
Laura Terrill
Annie Toomes
Vivian Tremaine, R.R.C.
Nellie Tuck
Frances Upton, A.R.R.C.
Lottie Urquhart, M.M.
Christina M. Watling, A.R.R.C.
Fanny L. Walker
Rose Wall
Everetta Watters
Marjorie Webb, A.R.R.C.
Eveline Whitney, A.R.R.C.
Sarah E. Young, A.R.R.C.

WORLD WAR II — 1939-1945

Mary A. Abbott
R. Catherine Aikin
F. Moyra Allen
Verna C. Andrews
Julia Andrews
Catherine G. Angus
Dorothea R. Atkinson
Barbara C. Baird
Barbara M. Bamford
Luise H. Baptist
Dorothy R. Barclay
Lois M. Bayly
Elizabeth B. Beaugrand
Jessie I. Bell
Meredith W. Bennett
Evelyn R. Berens
Muriel S. Betts
Phyllis I. Bishop
Beatrice E. Black
M. Jean Blackler
Mary E. Bray, M.I.D.
Jessie Bresse
E. Amelia Brown
Helen M. Brown
Mary T. Brown
May K. Bunbury
Dorothy M. Burgess
Lily M. Burri
Margaret A. Burrow
Mary D. Burt
Frances Callanan
Phyllis C. Cameron
Martha B. Campbell
Grace S. Carter
Margot P. Carson
Elizabeth L. Cavers
Marguerite A. Cerat
Gladys L. Chaplin
Helen Christian
Marion E. Chute
Mary Clarke
Joan D. Clarkson
Alison C. Cleland
Margaret E. Clunie
Christine M. Cole
Dorothy R. Colquhoun
Hazel M. Coolican
Elaine M. Cornish
Pauline Cox
Winnifred Crombie
Anne E. Cromwell, A.R.R.C.
Irene C. Cunningham
F. Margaret Dakin
Eleanor F. Davis
Kathleen Derby
Patricia C. DeMerrall
Matilda M. Devere
Ella V. Dixon
C. Elaine Doherty
Joan M. Dorning
Alix E. Doull
Barbara R. Eardley-Wilmot
Lorna J. Ellard
Evelyn S. Elliott
Florence S. Evans
Margaret L. Fairweather
Robina S. Falls
Madeline E. Farmer, M.I.D.
Margaret A. Farquhar
Jessie A. Fawthrop
Constance B. Findlay
Geraldine B. Fitzgerald
E. Doreen Flannigan
Mary A. Fleming
Alma C. Fletcher
Irene C. Fraser

Thelma H. Fuller
Margaret l. Fulton
Katherine E. Gardner
Isabel D. Gibson
Joan L. Gray
Edith F. Groundwater
Marguerite J. Hall
Helen G. Hamilton
Frances H. Hanchet
Mabel Mae Harper
Margaret E. Harrison
Agnes B. Hass
Kathleen N. Hayward
Katherine L. Hebb
Ida Henderson, R.R.C. (2nd Class,
Blanche G. Herman, R.R.C. (1st Class)—M.I.D.
Helen G. Hewton, A.R.R.C.
H. Teresa Hickman
Elizabeth A. Hodgson
K. Evlyn Horsfall
Margaret A. Howard
Audrey E. Hunter
Eileen Ingram
Helen G. Irving
Mary Irving
Jane C. Jacobs
Doris A. Jamieson
Annie P. Johnson
Doreen B. Johnson
Isabel E. Johnston
Bertha A. Johnstone
Marie M. Kelly
Nancy B. Kennedy-Reid, R.R.C. (1st Class)
Katherine H. Kindle
Elsie P. King
Miriam King
Beatrice W. Kinnear
Rowena P. Kitchen
Jean Knecht
Alide O. Knowlton
Esme S. Labreque
Gertrude E. Lake
Isabel M. Lamplough
Edith F. Langley
Shirley M. Laughlin
Adoree W. Lebrooy
Edith C. Little
Hilaire Little
Vera M. Maile
Adelene J. Martinello
Francis Melkman, R.R.C.
Mary Ellen Morrison
A. Mary Morrison
Margaret C. Moss
Olive V. Mulligan
Dorothy E. Murphy, A.R.R.C.
Isobel M. Murphy
Catherine S. Murray, A.R.R.C.
Theodora MacDonald
Cecil M. MacDonald, A.R.R.C. DSM (Greece)
Eileen V. MacDonald
Florence J. MacDonald
Jeanette M. MacDonald
Ruth A. MacDonald
Margaret M. MacDonald
Isabel N. MacIver
Marjorie S. MacLean
Katrine C. MacLeod
Marguerite E. MacLeod
Janet E. MacNearney
Edith MacQuiston
Dorothy I. MacRae, R.R.C. (1st Class)
Janet K. MacRae
Vivienne M. MacRae
Myrtle M. MacTavish
Margaret J. McCann, M.B.E.

Mary M. McCarthy
Eileen G. McCready
Olga M. McCrudden
Thirza M. McCullough
Mary C. McDermott
Phyllis T. McElroy
Emma McEwen
Katherine McKim
Catherine S. McLeister
Hilda B. McLeod
Isabel M. McLeod
Edith W. McOuat
Helen E. McQueen
Constance Norris
Rosamund W. Neill
Mary Louise Newton
Louise E. O'Hara
Mary A. O'Regan
Beatrice E. Owen
A. Mary Pae
Clara A. Partington
Jean L. Parsons
Muriel G. Paterson
Jeannette M. Paul
Lilian E. Payn
Ethyle I. Percival
Monica V. Perram
Pearl S. Phillips
Muriel N. Pope
Julia G. Pugh
Phyllis M. Reay
Eleanor N. Reid
Doretta J. Reid
Elizabeth F. Ross
Jean C. Ross
Jeannette M. Savard
Emma C. Schroeder
Marjorie D. Schryer
Elizabeth M. Scott
Ruth Scott, M.I.D.
Helen K. Shaw
Miriam A. Shaw
Louise M. Shepherd

Norma B. Siddons-Gray
Muriel E. Small
Grace A. Smeaton
Amy K. Smith
Elizabeth A. Smith
Margaret Smith
Margaret C. Snider
Williamina C. Spence
Ethel E. Starkey
Olive I.. Stewart
Dorothy M. Surgenor
Mary F.. Sykes
Madeline S. Taylor, M.I.D.
Dorothy A. Templeman
Agnes I. Tennant, R.R.C.
L. Elizabeth Tennant
Barbara J. Thomas
Phyllis E. Thomas
May L. Thomson
Anne Thorpe
May E. Tracey-Gould
Marjorie M. Tupper
Charlotte W. Turner
Verna R. Umphrey
Maria E. Van Bommell
Margaret E. Van Scoyoc
Gladys M. Vass
Kathleen A. Walker
Phyllis E. Walker
V. Ruth Walker
Gertrude A. Wallace
Edythe Ward
Mary Ward
Jennie B. Wareham
Doris V. Watson
Margaret J. Watt
Hilda R. Welling
Mildred K. Wilbur
Doris E. Wilson
Gweneth L. Woodburn
Elaine S. Wright
Mary R. Yelland

149

INDEX

Abbott, Dr. Maude, ii, 117
Admission age, 80
Admission books, early, 7
Alexander, Charles, 18, 25
Alexandra Hospital, 68, 75
Alcoholic stimulants, 5; suggested
    reduction in, 16
Alumnae Association, formation of,
    114; Reunion, ii, 73
Anniversary of Training School, 115
Archibald, H., 15
Arnton, J. J., 15

Baikie, Miss, 44, 117
Basic nursing, 75
Basic sciences, place of, 74
Bazin, A. T., 50, 120
Beer, allowance of, 3
Bethune, Strachan, 16
Binmore, Chas., 15
Birkett, H. S., 101, 120
Blackader, A. D., 104
Blackwood, Dr., 7
Bland, Mrs., 7
Bleeding basins, 5
Blower, Miss, 24
Bolster, Miss J., 120
Browne, Miss M., 115
Bush, Miss A., 117
Buzzell, Miss G., 64

Caldwell, Wm., 2, 7
Campbell, G. W., 27
Carbolic spray, 121
Carmichael, H. B., 108
Carroll, Miss G., 45
Catherine Booth Hospital, 75
Chapel, arrangements for, 30
Chapman, Miss E., 45
Cholera, epidemic of, 7
Christie, Miss Anna, i, 76
Cline, J., 26
Closse, Lambert, 2
Club, Graduate Nurses', 114
Colley, Miss G., 120
Collins, Miss M., 119
Collyer, Miss, 40, 44
Colquhoun, Miss A., 116
Committee of Management, origin, 1
Como, Que., 36
Contagious diseases, 119
Cookery, teaching of, 42
Cooper, Miss E., 119
Cotter, Father, 62
Course of training, original, 53
Craik, R., 13
Crawford, J., 16
Critical Survey of School, 76
Curriculum, changes in, 74; survey of, 75
Curriculum Committee, 76

Davis, Miss, 119
Day, J. J., 26
Deadhouse, complaints about, 15
Denniston, Miss M. J., 79

Denovan, Miss C., 59
Department Veterans' Affairs, 78
Diagnoses, 2
Diet kitchen, original location of, 43
Discharging of nurses, 11
Discipline of nurses, 40
Drains, overhauling of, 101
Draper, Miss E. A., 36
Dunfield, Mrs., 120
Dunlop, Miss H., 116, 118
Dunne, Miss A., 34, 45, 49 *seq.*, 117, 119

Eberts, E. M., ii, 114
England, E., 117
English, Miss J., 45
Evans, D. J., 94

Female Benevolent Society, 1
Fenwick, G. E., 4
Flies, annoyance from, 15
Flynn, Mrs., 4
Finley, F. G., 35, 120
Fire hazard in hospital, 6
Fire in hospital, 109
First graduates, 45
Forbes, Miss, 17

Garbage tins near wards, 15
Gas first used, 6
Gerrard, Samuel, 2
Gibb, Mrs. B., 1
Gilday, Lorne, C., 77
Gordon, Keith, 57
Graduate Nurses' Club, 114
Graduation ceremonies, 46; revival
    of, 63
Graduation of first class, 47
Graduate nurses in private pavilion,
    67; in wards, 64
Gray, James, 31
Greatorex, Mrs., 44
Group dynamics, 76

Hamilton, Hubert, 92, 119
Hamilton, W. F., 120
Henderson, Mrs. J., 120
Herman, Miss Blanche, 72
Hersey, Miss Viola, 119, 120
Hetherington, Miss C., 117
Holmes, A. F., 2
Holt, Miss Mabel, 55, 63, 76; appointed
    supt., 66
Honor Rolls, 77
Hoskins, Eliz., 12
Hospital, early life in, 3; additions to,
    14; inspection by English nurses, 18;
    cost of running, 19; inadequacy of,
    23; conditions in 1881, 29; unsatis-
    factory conditions in, 33; Miss
    Livingston's description of, 39;
    moving of, 71
Hotel Dieu, 1
Hours of duty, 80
House of Recovery, 1, 83
Housing of nurses, 64

150